Living with Breast Cancer

A Guide for Facilitating Self-Help Groups

Pat Kelly and PISCES
Partners in Self-Help Community
Education and Support

The Susan G. Komen
Breast Cancer Foundation

2000
B.C. Decker Inc.
Hamilton

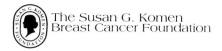
Y-me National Breast Cancer Organization℠

B.C. Decker Inc.
20 Hughson St. South
P.O. Box 620, L.C.D. 1
Hamilton, Ontario L8N 3K7
Tel: 905-522-7017; Fax: 905-522-7839
Email: info@bcdecker.com
Website: www.bcdecker.com

00 01 02 03 /PC/ 9 8 7 6 5 4 3 2 1
ISBN 1-896998-07-0

Sales and Distribution

United States
B.C. Decker Inc.
P.O. Box 785
Lewiston, NY 14092-0785
Tel: 905-522-7017 / 1-800-568-7281
Fax: 905-522-7839
E-mail: info@bcdecker.com
Website: www.bcdecker.com

Canada
B.C. Decker Inc.
20 Hughson Street South
P.O. Box 620, L.C.D. 1
Hamilton, Ontario L8N 3K7
Tel: 905-522-7017 / 1-800-568-7281
Fax: 905-522-7839
E-mail: info@bcdecker.com
Website: www.bcdecker.com

UK, Europe, Scandinavia, Middle East
Harcourt Publishers Limited
Customer Service Department
Foots Cray High Street
Sidcup, Kent
DA14 5HP, UK
Tel: 44 (0) 208 308 5760
Fax: 44 (0) 181 308 5702
E-mail: cservice@harcourt_brace.com

Japan
Igaku-Shoin Ltd.
Foreign Publications Department
3-24-17 Hongo
Bunkyo-ku, Tokyo, Japan 113-8719
Tel: 3 3817 5680
Fax: 3 3815 6776
E-mail: fd@igaku.shoin.co.jp

Singapore, Malaysia, Thailand,
Philippines, Indonesia, Vietnam,
Pacific Rim
Harcourt Asia Pte Limited
583 Orchard Road
#09/01, Forum
Singapore 238884
Tel: 65-737-3593
Fax: 65-753-2145

Foreign Rights
John Scott & Company
International Publishers' Agency
P.O. Box 878
Kimberton, PA 19442
Tel: 610-827-1640
Fax: 610-827-1671

Notice: This guide has been designed to be used by laypersons conducting
breast cancer survivor support groups. We believe that properly structured
and conducted support groups can be of great comfort and assistance to survivors as they cope with the unique emotional and physical issues that they
face. It is important to note, however, that this manual is not intended, nor
should it be used, as a substitute for professional medical or psychological
care. Accordingly, all survivors should maintain communication with a quali-
fied medical professional on a regular basis.

Printed in Canada

Dear Friends:

On behalf of the Susan G. Komen Breast Cancer Foundation, I would like to thank you for your interest in developing and providing a support program for women facing breast cancer. As a breast cancer survivor, I know that there is no greater tool for fighting this disease than the power of shared human resources.

The Komen Foundation is so proud to have played a role in the development of this unique manual. Collaborating on this project with Y-ME and PISCES has been extremely rewarding and has resulted in a powerful resource for those starting a breast cancer support group and for groups that already exist. Being written by and for women living with breast cancer makes this manual exceptional and unique and demonstrates the true meaning of "caring by sharing."

I started the Komen Foundation in 1982 to honor the memory of my sister Suzy, who died of breast cancer at the age of 36. Shortly before she died, I promised her that I would do everything I could to help women so that they would not have to go through what she did. Back then, women didn't talk about breast cancer; today, it is an open topic of conversation. It is no longer a death sentence; more women than ever are living wonderfully full lives following a diagnosis. Thanks to collaborative efforts like the development of this resource, women's lives have been saved and their quality of life improved.

But a resource can only be helpful if it is used. Thank you for making this manual come to life and for encouraging women to share their experience, strength, and hope. You are truly making a difference in the lives of many!

Sincerely,
Nancy Brinker
Founding Chair
The Susan G. Komen
Breast Cancer Foundation

Background

> Never doubt that a small group of concerned, committed citizens can change the world; indeed it is the only thing that ever has.
>
> MARGARET MEAD

Today, there are about 2 million women living in the United States who have been diagnosed with breast cancer. Each and every year another 180,000 American women are told, "I'm sorry, but you have breast cancer." More and more, these women and their families are turning to self-help groups to find the comfort, support, and information they need to learn to live with cancer. This manual has been written for them and by them, to offer help to other women who are starting and leading breast cancer self-help groups.

Three organizations that are familiar with the challenges faced by breast cancer survivors partnered in the production of this manual. They are:

- **The Susan G. Komen Breast Cancer Foundation**. Working with local Affiliates and Komen Race for the Cure® events across the country, the Komen Foundation is fighting to eradicate breast cancer as a life-threatening disease. In addition to funding research, the Foundation funds education, screening, and treatment projects in communities from coast to coast and delivers the life-saving message of early detection to hundreds of thousands of women and men.

- **The Y-ME National Breast Cancer Organization**. Since its simple beginnings around a kitchen table in 1978, Y-ME volunteers and staff have been providing telephone information and support, along with a national network of Y-ME chapters that provide self-help group meetings and public education programs.

- **PISCES — Partnering In Self-Help Community Education & Support**. Since 1987, Pat Kelly, PISCES President and breast cancer survivor, has been working with local and national cancer patient groups to provide skills training and development.

Purpose

The most exciting and powerful capability of self-help groups is that ordinary people can start them in their local communities when none currently exist, and then go on to provide extraordinary help to others. These group founders don't require a government grant, an agency, endowment or office—just the inspiration and help from a few other people who share the concern and interest.[1]

Living with Breast Cancer: A Guide for Facilitating Self-Help Groups was written to offer encouragement and ideas to women involved with breast cancer self-help groups and to help those who are just getting started. The information about starting and maintaining a breast cancer group has been developed from research and published reports about self-help and support groups and from the skills and experiences of the members of the Project Advisory Committee.

The main purpose of a breast cancer group is to provide a safe, welcoming place for women to both give and receive support. Groups can lose sight of their goal of providing support and help when they undertake fundraising or outreach programs or newsletters. What your group members decide they are able to do and what they want to do are the things your group SHOULD do.

---

[1] *The Self-Help Sourcebook.* 6th Ed. Denville, NJ: American Self-Help Clearinghouse, 1998.

How to Use This Guide

If you are just getting started, you may want to read the manual from cover to cover to give you some ideas. You can go through the chapters in order or you can read through the Table of Contents and find what looks most interesting to you. Read that section first, then go on to the rest as needed. If your group is already up and running, you might use a highlighter and mark what is helpful.

In the back of the manual you will find a section on research about self-help and a list of resources. We have also included stories and quotations from women who are involved with groups to illustrate the ideas in the text so that you might remember the suggestions when you face similar situations.

This guide is intended to help answer your questions and give some direction, but you and your group members are the best people to decide how to make your group work. The most helpful way for you to learn how to facilitate group meetings will come from "just doing it."

Acknowledgments

This guide builds upon the lessons learned from breast cancer self-help and support groups across America. In gratitude and appreciation, we thank the members of the Project Advisory Committee for generously giving their time and effort in bringing this work to you:

David Cella, PhD
Director of the Center on Outcomes,
Research and Education
Evanston Northwestern Healthcare
Evanston, IL

Linda L. Frame, RN, MS, AOCN
Director of Education
The Susan G. Komen Breast Cancer Foundation
Dallas, TX

Beverly Rogers
Director of Chapter Services
Y-ME National Breast Cancer Organization
Chicago, IL

Crystal Walsh, MSW
Vice Chair, Education
The Susan G. Komen Breast Cancer Foundation
Dallas, TX

This publication was helped by a number of people who generously participated through telephone interviews, questionnaires, and reviewing drafts of the manual. We are most grateful for their contributions:

Ellie Lang, President
Y-ME of Central Indiana

Carol Forhan, Past President
Y-ME Ladies of Courage, California

Elaine S. Hill, Founder and President
Y-ME of Chattanooga
Tennessee

Lorna Patrick
The Mary-Helen Mautner Project
for Lesbians with Cancer
Washington, DC

Barbara Oliver,
Executive Director
Y-ME of Connecticut

Betty Kaiser, President
Y-ME of Arizona

Catherine Traiforou
Gilda's Club, New York
New York

Catalino Ramos,
Director of Special Populations
Y-ME, National Breast Cancer
Organization, Chicago, IL

Joal Fischer, MD
Executive Director
SupportWorks
Charlotte, NC

Diana Rowden
The Susan G. Komen Breast
Cancer Foundation
Dallas, TX

Photographs courtesy of:
Lottie Grant
Nancy Fox
Vi McIsaac
Jackie Miller
Oakville Chapter
Breast Cancer Support Services

Stock Photography courtesy of:
Page 13: ©Owen Franken/CORBIS/Magma Photo News
Page 34: ©Ron Chapple/Masterfile
Page 36: ©Dennis Degnan/CORBIS/MAGMA
Page 42: ©Joel W. Rogers/CORBIS/MAGMA
Page 52: ©Dick Luria/Masterfile
Page 62: ©James P. Blair/CORBIS/MAGMA
Page 72: ©Jim Whitmer/Masterfile
Page 79: © Layne Kennedy/CORBIS/MAGMA
Page 82: ©Dick Luria/Masterfile
Page 87: ©Bill Brooks/Masterfile
Page 95: ©Leif Skoogfors/CORBIS/MAGMA

Table of Contents

CHAPTER 1

What Is Self-Help?

What you can expect to learn about in this chapter:
- Understanding what self-help is.
- Common topics in group.
- Four ways groups help members.
- Working with professionals.

On a recent Thursday, about a dozen women met in the church parlor as they have every Thursday since January. As they entered the room, snapping shut umbrellas, shaking rain off their raincoats, they were already talking full speed. One told about her grandchild, due 10 days ago, but still not born. Another brought in gifts she'd made for a friend, which everyone admired. Still another brought in cookies and a bottle of apple cider. There was nothing unusual in the way they greeted each other, laughed together and settled into a circle to talk. They were like any other group of women getting together for an evening.

The truth is that these women have known each other less than 10 months—and what they have in common is that each of them has, at some point, sat in a doctor's office while the doctor said the words, "You have breast cancer."

And that, they agree among themselves, was one of those moments in time when you suddenly know that everything in the world has changed for you—and that, whatever happens, you can never go back to the way things were before.[2]

---

[2]"Only They Know." Sandi Kahn, New Haven Register, October 18, 1998. Reproduced with permission.

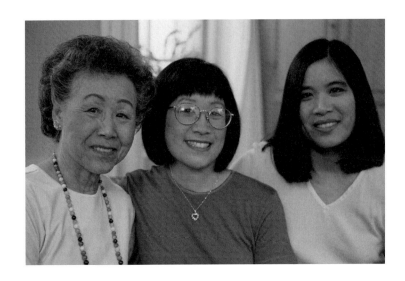

What Is a Breast Cancer Self-Help Group All About?

Self-Help happens when people who share a common problem come together to help each other. At hospitals and cancer centers, women receive the medical care they need to treat their disease. At breast cancer self-help groups, women learn what they need to know to live with breast cancer; they learn to find hope and how to cope with the diagnosis. Groups create a safe, welcoming place for those who are struggling with this illness to talk, find information about treatments, and give support and encouragement to others.

What Do Members Talk About?

In preparing to write this guide, we talked with breast cancer survivors* from groups across the United States. These women told us about feeling "out of control" and powerless when they first learned they had breast cancer. Joining a self-help group has helped many to regain self-confidence and begin to plan for the future. Again and again, women talked about the need for information and the need to meet others living with breast cancer because other survivors symbolize hope. In all of these groups, there was a common bond of belonging to a group where they didn't need to explain—where every member had a cancer story.

---

*The author is using the definition of cancer survivor provided by the National Coalition for Cancer Survivorship: anyone with a history of cancer from the point of diagnosis and for the remainder of life.

Living with Breast Cancer

Women in breast cancer groups often discuss personal struggles in marriages or partnerships, sexuality, dependency, loneliness, and difficulty talking with family, friends, and doctors. Other concerns include:

- Fear of death or pain,
- Coping with treatment decisions and side effects,
- Relationships with doctors and other health care providers,
- Complementary therapies, and
- Financial and insurance problems.

Being able to share stories, talk about problems, and express strong emotions creates an important bond. The sense of relief that comes from bonding is an important part of group effectiveness. These are the emotions that are often withheld from family and other loved ones because we feel a need to protect them from our fears about cancer. In groups, we find a safe place to speak about these feelings and let them go. Finally, breast cancer groups can be a safe place to confront our fears and to learn new ways of being.

How are Groups Helpful to Members?

Shirley told about a secret fear she had during chemotherapy that the medicine wasn't working because her hair wasn't falling out, as she expected. "I worried and worried to myself about this, and then Cindy joined the group, and she hadn't lost her hair either—and it was so important to me to know that, I mean I was SO relieved."

People in self-help groups talk about helping one another in four ways:

1. By listening and telling one another their stories (peer support).

2. By sharing information, education, and experience.

3. By giving emotional support and modeling coping skills.

4. By helping create a sense of belonging to the group.

For the women coming to groups, the help they find must fit with the kind of help they need in order to be effective. If someone is seeking information and finds a group meeting focused only on talking about feelings, that person won't feel satisfied. Ask new people who are coming for the first time what kinds of help they expect to find.

Knowing that members share a range of problems in common can provide some sense of comfort. It will also be more likely that your group is able to meet the needs of members when those needs are clearly expressed. Having a balanced focus on education or information and informal discussion will help to keep meetings meaningful.

People want to feel better, and they believe that talking with people who are going through or have gone through cancer treatment will help. Although these expectations are not always met, most support groups satisfy the need for comfort and connection with others who share a similar experience. Again, women who are disappointed or anxious with the intensity, intimacy, or frank discussions will probably leave the group because it frightens them or doesn't meet their expectations.

The goal for the group is to provide encouragement and reinforcement to members, to show respect for each member and her choices, to share information, and to discuss ways of coping.

What Are the Benefits of Joining a Breast Cancer Group?

My patients have found self-help groups to be very helpful; they often feel that unless you have had cancer, one cannot truly understand.

FAMILY DOCTOR

The most important feature of self-help is that the person giving help and the person receiving help are equals, and everyone in the group can do both. Finding that others have the same or similar problems helps group members to feel they are no longer alone. Here are some of the other benefits that people in cancer support groups have talked about:

- Learning more about breast cancer and treatment options;
- Learning about available resources such as books, tapes, and other kinds of groups;
- Feeling that life is more meaningful;
- Being better able to cope with illness and medical procedures;
- Feeling less fearful;
- Being more able to talk about cancer;
- Being more able to talk with family and friends;
- Feeling stronger;
- Feeling better able to make choices;
- Being less alone or lonely; and
- Being more active.

In groups, women can tell their story in an honest and direct way and, at the same time, learn from the stories other women tell about living with this disease. Together group members clarify problems and think through possible solutions. Long-time members often become mentors or coaches for newly diagnosed patients. By learning how other people have coped with similar experiences, we can help newly diagnosed women to cut through some of the confusion and regain strength and hope.

> I wholeheartedly believe in self-help groups and feel that our local cancer group is invaluable.
>
> FAMILY DOCTOR

Even when members experience recurrence of their disease and when members die, other members report learning powerful lessons about healing. As difficult and frightening as it may seem for someone just starting a new group, talking and learning from other people who are living with cancer can be strengthening and rewarding.

There is also strong evidence that people who have social support—such as family, friends, coworkers, self-help groups—are healthier than those who do not. Research has demonstrated that people who have strong social and family structures are less anxious and less depressed. In this manual you will find information about some of the current research on the benefits of cancer self-help groups (Appendix B).

What Makes a Cancer Self-Help Group Effective?

A group is working well when it can meet members' needs. A second way in which groups work depends on whether members are satisfied with their relationships with other members. This is important for group cohesion. When members find others who have learned to cope and begin to find new meaning in their own life, they value the group in a new way.

A third way that groups work is when members feel proud about the work they are doing together. A group culture develops in which women feel a bond of intimacy, commitment, acceptance,

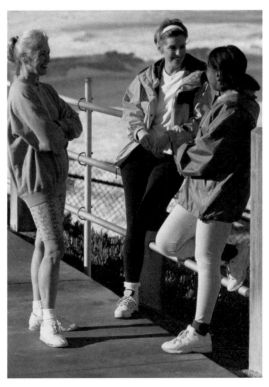

Living with Breast Cancer

understanding, and safety. Members can derive satisfaction purely from belonging to the group. Last, many women describe a good group meeting as one where there has been a lot of laughter. Laughter seems to provide relief from the struggles with cancer and treatments.

Finally, one of the challenges for successful cancer groups and other self-help groups is to recognize the limits of what can be done. People who are suicidal, clinically depressed, or suffering from serious mental illness need professional medical help. A self-help group can help to direct people to find out about the appropriate resources. In this way, a self-help group becomes part of a continuum of care that responds according to individual needs without trying to fill everyone's needs.

How Are Self-Help Groups Different from Professionally Led Groups?

The following chart explains different types of groups.

Group Type	Focus	Facilitator
Self-help	• Common characteristics or concerns • Mutual support	Peer facilitator
Support and/or education	• Information and support • Ability to address complexity of psychosocial issues and coping strategies beyond mutual support	Mental health professional, health care professional, or group member with formal training in group dynamics
Therapy	• Individual change as a result of group experience	Mental health professional

Generic group definition: "Any network of persons with some common identified need who meet regularly to exchange information and share common experiences." Adapted from Man to Man Facilitator Training Manual (American Cancer Society).

Self-help groups are different from other kinds of groups mainly because the person helping and the person being helped are equal members of the group. The self-help group facilitator shares the common problem of other members. In contrast, a therapy group is usually led by a professional such as a social worker or psychologist, and the group meetings are often sponsored by a hospital or national organization. Although there are differences, what is more important is what these groups have in common: members learning from other cancer survivors and finding hope and healing through shared experiences.

Whether the group uses a self-help model or a professionally led model, the facilitator's role is to promote discussion in a safe environment, provide information, remind members of agreements, and assist when there are problems. An effective facilitator helps the group to function in a safe, welcoming manner.

How Can Self-Helpers and Helping Professionals Work Together?

Over time, as self-help has become recognized and credible in its own right, groups are becoming more comfortable working in partnership with professionals. A number of self-help groups want to have professionals involved, included as co-facilitators. The benefits of participation from professionals is supported by research that shows that active involvement, such as helping groups get started, consulting, and presenting, improves linkages with self-helpers and strengthens the effectiveness of both self-help and professional approaches.

I think one of the things we did right early on was that we made a big effort to gain the confidence of the doctors and that is really crucial in starting a group because they are protective of their patients. And we had to assure them first of all that we were serious about what we were doing and our purpose was to help. That we weren't selling anything or any point of view and that we would not be interfering in the treatment of their patients. And the fact that we have a high-quality program.

One way of finding the right mix of professional involvement is a partnership agreement built on flexibility, respect, understanding, and shared goals. Professionals can and do make valuable contributions to groups, however, their roles should not cause group members to be overwhelmed by the authority of the professional.

As a simple guideline, the expression "on tap, not on top" may help to define the right partnership between self-helpers and professional helpers.

KEY MESSAGES FROM THIS CHAPTER:

- The authority or credibility of a cancer self-help group is built on the belief that people who share a common problem have expertise that comes from living with the problem.

- Members of a cancer self-help group both give and receive support.

- Groups provide a sense of optimism and hope for healing.

- Self-help groups and professionals can work together to meet members' needs.

CHAPTER 2

Before You Start A Group

A self-help group can be started by anyone with a bit of courage, a sense of committment, and a good dose of caring.

ED MADARA, DIRECTOR OF THE AMERICAN SELF-HELP CLEARINGHOUSE

What you can expect to learn about in this chapter:
- **History of three breast cancer groups.**
- **Training that helps you to start a group.**
- **Principles of self-help.**
- **How to find others who share your vision.**
- **Common stages of group development.**

History of Three Breast Cancer Groups

ARIZONA

The network started in 1991. We hold monthly education meetings and a rap session and we operate a hotline. We generally have a physician or other medical personnel come and talk for an hour and then we have a question and answer time and then we have a facilitator that leads the group discussion. It was started by a couple of women with breast cancer. They just felt that nobody should face breast cancer alone and they were also into advocacy for funding for research.

WASHINGTON, DC

Our group started to provide a safe place where lesbians can be with each other and support themselves through their treatment so that they don't feel alone and so that they have at least one place where they can go and be surrounded by people like them and who understand their special issues. Lesbians have loving relationships that they want to bring into their healing process. It is not as easy as when a man is your partner. There is just so much anxiety around coming out during your illness. Because just like everybody else they want their partner there and I think that is one of the main issues—it causes anxiety because you never really know how people are going to react to you. It is the last thing you need at this particular time in your life—to have your partner at home because they can't be part of your illness or treatment or healing.

CALIFORNIA
There were six women who got together around the kitchen table. They decided they wanted more than just talking to each other about their problems, even though their problems were similar. We all have breast cancer, but we all had different treatments, and why is that? Why are you taking that and I'm not? So the six women decided they wanted to start a group for information and education.

From these examples, you can see that the ways in which breast cancer groups get started are as different as the women involved. Most of the women who start groups admit that the beginnings are both exciting and difficult. There is no magic formula for success. Understanding that self-help groups work best when they are small, informal, warm, and safe might help you to feel less overwhelmed at the start. Thankfully, the basic practices of the self-help movement describe a very simple and effective place to begin.[3]

- Be brave.
- Start small.
- Use what you've got.
- Do something you enjoy.
- Don't overcommit.

[3] Dass R, Bush M. *Compassion in Action: Setting Out on the Path of Service.* New York, NY: Bell Tower Books, 1992:174.

Do I Need Special Training to Start a Self-Help Group?

You don't need special training, nor do you need to be an expert or a professional to start a self-help group. Your compassion and willingness to work and share your experiences will be your most important assets in the beginning. Your skills and confidence will grow over time as you learn to facilitate meetings.

You might want to start by taking stock of your group skills. This manual has a worksheet called <u>A Personal Skills Inventory</u>. (Appendix A). You can use the worksheet to help you identify the

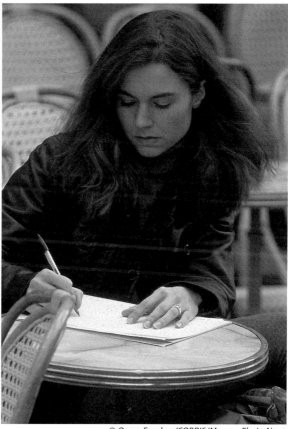

© Owen Franken/CORBIS/Magma Photo News

specific skills you already have for facilitating teams and groups and to identify the areas where you need to practice or increase your skills.

How Can I Find Other Women Who Are Interested in a Breast Cancer Support Group?

CHECK OUT EXISTING GROUPS

Don't reinvent the wheel. Chances are pretty good that a breast cancer group already exists in your community or nearby. If there is a local self-help clearinghouse serving your area, call to find out about other groups (American Self-Help Clearinghouse, Appendix D). Contact the national offices of breast cancer organizations listed in the Resources section of this manual to find out if they have nearby chapters that can help you. Ask about self-help groups or facilitators nearest to you and think about calling them. Find out if you can attend their meetings to get a feel for how they work.

Think about sharing the work and the rewards, right from the start, if you are starting a new group. Look for other women who share your experience and some of your values. Working with others will help when the workload grows and it will help keep *you* from burning out.

ADVERTISE

Circulate a flyer or letter that specifically asks that if "you are interested in joining with others to help start a breast cancer group" they should contact you. Include your first name, telephone number, and time and place for the meeting. Post the copies where you think it is appropriate. Mail copies to key people. Ask if the notice can be published in your local paper.

FORM AN ORGANIZING COMMITTEE

When you get responses from women who are interested in starting a group, ask about their interests and what they would like the group to do. Ask if they are willing to share the responsibilities of organizing the first group meetings for a period of time. Find out what group experiences or community efforts they are involved with. Arrange a convenient time to bring this small group together to get to know one another, start sharing ideas, and plan for the first meeting.

But, most important, when you have your first meeting and start sending out messages about what you are doing, it will be seen as a group effort and not just one person.

TIPS

✔ *Ask the people you met at the cancer treatment center, clinic, or hospital. Other patients, nurses, and oncologists might be able to help or they may know someone else who is interested.*

✔ *Nurses and office staff who work with breast surgeons see many women when they are newly diagnosed. They can be very helpful in referring women to your group. Talk to them about what you are planning and start building good relationships.*

✔ *Talk about your ideas with family, friends, coworkers, and neighbors. Leave your name and contact number with people who will pass it along.*

✔ *Post a notice at the clinic, hospital, or treatment center. Health food stores, the YMCA or YWCA, and wellness centers are places that cancer patients and survivors also look for information. Ask if you can post notices in these places.*

✔ *Talk to other self-help group leaders in your community, especially other women's health groups or other cancer groups.*

✔ *Call the local offices or chapters of established cancer organizations and charities; ask if they have self-help services or training workshops. Tell them what you are looking for and ask how you can work together.*

✔ *Family doctors are another source for referring patients and they need to know what you are planning and how to contact your group.*

✔ *Don't be too discouraged if others don't share your enthusiasm. Remember that this is a group for breast cancer patients and survivors. Patients and survivors often have different views from other people about their needs for support. If you are convinced that there is a need for a group, you will find other women with breast cancer who share your vision soon enough. Don't give up.*

Creating a Place for Diversity

Some of the challenges and rewards of working in cancer groups come from learning about different cultures, different beliefs, and different life experiences.

Points of difference:

- Thoughts about why people get sick, why we get cancer, and how people get well;
- Beliefs about the role of health professionals and health practices in healing;
- Attitudes about our bodies;
- Past experience with illness;
- Ideas about suffering, pain, and loss;
- Different ideas about support, families, friends, professionals, and institutions;
- Ways of caring and understanding who is responsible for caring;
- How we feel about asking for support;
- Ways of communicating and expressing emotions;
- Ways of working in groups;
- Ideas about what is okay to talk about and what isn't; and
- Understanding the unique health needs of women.

If you want your support group to be welcoming to all, you will need to involve women from a variety of backgrounds and experiences. Women at various stages of diagnosis and treatment will have different perspectives. Lesbians and women who partner with women, those who are younger or older, and women from diverse cultures and backgrounds will bring a range of experiences that will enrich your group culture.

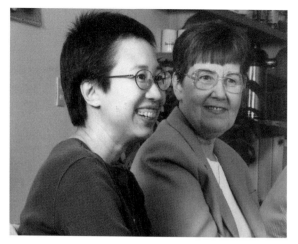

There are also groups specifically for different groups of women with breast cancer. Lesbians, Latins, African-American women, and younger women have all started separate breast cancer groups. There are groups especially for women with recurrence, and the members seem to prefer to meet separately, at least for part of their group time. Other subgroups join with a larger group for part of their meetings—usually the beginning and the end—then break off for a separate, small-group discussion. Again, the more we feel we share in common with other group members, the more comfortable and accepted we will feel and the less time we will spend explaining ourselves.

If your group pays attention to being welcoming and working to overcome barriers, newcomers will recognize your genuine intention to be supportive. Simple strategies such as serving refreshments or coordinating potluck meals have been suggested as events for generating interest around which self-help naturally happens. Overcoming barriers such as transportation to and from meetings or child care costs is important. To attract women from diverse communities, your group should identify issues that reflect the needs of those communities. One suggestion for a diverse group might be to talk about different approaches to overcoming the stigma of a cancer diagnosis and of asking for support. With older cancer patients and survivors, providing transportation, easy access for wheelchairs and walking aids, daytime meetings, allowing family members to attend, and programs with a specific topic would attract more people.

More important than our differences is what we share in common: the conviction that together we can overcome our loneliness and isolation.

Knowing the Stages of Group Development

You might find it helpful to know something about what might be on the journey up ahead as your group is getting started. In general, groups move in and out of various stages, and the behaviors described in the following chart can happen at any time. One of the jobs of the group facilitator is to recognize and monitor the stages or phases of group development. When a group first gets started, members often don't talk much. Knowing the stages of group development can be helpful for the facilitator in understanding that the members are just getting to know each other.

One simple model for group development identifies the phases of group life as follows:

STAGE	DEVELOPMENT TASKS	BEHAVIORS
FORMING	• Get acquainted • Define purpose • Lay ground rules	• Members are anxious • Watchful, quiet, uncertain • Group leans on the facilitator
STORMING	• Sort out differences • Learn how to overcome resistance • Learn how to build unity	• Conflict is evident • May be hostility and confusion • Common reactions may include comments such as "We never did this before."

STAGE	DEVELOPMENT TASKS	BEHAVIORS
NORMING	• Some understanding has been achieved through storming • Members are more trusting and accepting of other's ideas and opinions • Members are less dependent on the leader and take more responsibility for group behaviors • Stronger sense of group purpose	• Courtesy, caring, and harmony among members • Stronger sense of belonging among members • Members are more confident, focused on each other, not the facilitator • Commitment to agreements and goals
PERFORMING	• Norming stage continues to mature • Members take responsibility for process • Dependency on the facilitator is replaced by interependence on each other • Effective problem solving and conflict resolution	• Members try new strengths • Members feel accepted and part of something important • All members participate • Creativity and "risk taking" is high
LEAVING	Group comes to an end	Members should have a chance to: • Express feelings about the loss of the group • Remember successes • Identify problems • Hear from other members about what the group meant • Celebrate and say goodbye to others

From Tuckman B. *Stages of Group Development: Evaluating Programs*. Boston: Allyn and Bacon Inc., 1979.

Before You Start A Group

- You don't need to be an expert to start a group.
- Before you start, check out other local groups.
- Talk to health care providers about your ideas.
- Find others who share your vision and form an organizing committee.
- Create a place for diversity.
- Recognize that all groups go through various stages of development.

CHAPTER 3

How to Get Going and Stay on Track

What you can expect to learn about in this chapter:
- How to develop a mission statement.
- Defining the group purpose and goals.
- How to develop guidelines, ground rules, and agreements.
- Naming your group.
- Keeping a group record.
- Planning and publicizing group meetings.

In the old days, when neighbor women came together to sew quilts or preserve food, they not only got the job done, but they enjoyed the connectedness, the humor, and the giving and receiving of support. This tradition continues today as women gather in self-help groups to help each other deal with the problems they share.

The feeling you want in a support group is informal, safe, and caring. It is friendship and social support with a purpose. Sometimes, this spirit just happens. But most people involved with breast cancer support groups recommend balancing some kind of simple structure with flexibility and awareness of your group members' changing needs and energy.

One member of a breast cancer support group that didn't have a facilitator or guidelines about how the group would work described her experience:

> Women were just complaining and crying,
> and one person was talking for a long time.

Having an effective facilitator and a simple structure that helps keep the group focused on members' needs has been the mainstay for many groups. Again, there is no formula that will tell you what kind of structure works best. This chapter will give you some ideas about how your group can balance the need for open discussion with the need for a safe structure.

What Are the First Steps?

1. DEFINE THE PURPOSE FOR THE GROUP: CREATE A MISSION STATEMENT

Determining the purpose of meeting as a group will be one of the first decisions to make. A mission statement can help to define the goals and purpose. A breast cancer self-help group might have a mission statement such as "To provide emotional support and information to women in our community who are affected by breast cancer."

The mission or purpose:

- Shines as a guiding light, drawing people toward the group;
- Directs the members to stay focused on the goals and activities; and
- Helps prevent confusion as the group grows.

For example, if a group decides that its purpose is to offer education, new members will not expect socializing to be a major part of meetings. Defining the type of group lays the groundwork for all future decisions that the group will make. A clear purpose will define the type of group and make clear to potential members what the group is about.

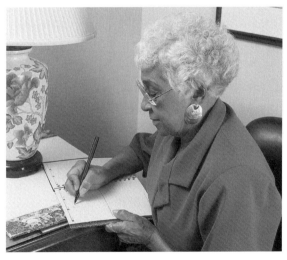

Living with Breast Cancer

2. Establish Goals

Once you decide the purpose, you will want to ensure that it is clearly understood by everyone, including new members. Often, groups will start every meeting by having a member of the group welcome everyone and explain the group's mission and purpose.

Once the purpose is clearly defined, group goals should be established. Goals emerge from the purpose and are usually stated as specific actions or activities of the group. One typical goal is to decrease the sense of isolation or loneliness that people with cancer often experience.

Groups can have many goals, including individual or personal goals and group goals. If you don't know what breast cancer patients and survivors in your community need from a group, you might want to have a discussion with the group about the goals they want, as part of the first group meeting.

Personal goals might include:

- Dealing with loneliness, fear, and isolation;
- Finding a unique kind of support;
- Sharing experiences with others who are similarly affected;
- Sharing information about services available;
- Providing a safe place to express feelings;
- Developing coping skills; and
- Increasing self-esteem.

Group goals might include:

- Learning from one another and providing encouragement;
- Developing coping skills;
- Sharing problem-solving strategies;
- Overcoming the stigma of a cancer diagnosis;

- Providing a focus when we feel confused and don't know where to begin;
- Exploring nontraditional resources;
- Helping members gain a sense of control;
- Providing relief for families and caregivers;
- Providing a safe, trusting, accepting, and confidential place;
- Raising awareness in the community about the needs of cancer survivors;
- Being a breast cancer information/education resource in the community; and
- Public speaking by members.

Your group may find it helpful to discuss some of these goals and how they might apply to your breast cancer group. These goals may also be helpful when you are describing your group to outsiders or when you are publishing a newsletter or flyers or posters that advertise your group.

A warning about goals: you don't need to do all of these or even any of them. You might choose to focus on one or two or none at all. Never pressure anyone to commit to anything more than attending and respecting the guidelines.

From time to time, when members are evaluating the effectiveness of the group, it may help to question if the purpose, needs, or expectations have changed. Members should be aware of changing needs and opportunities that come along and be prepared to respond to them.

3. Guidelines, Ground Rules, and Agreements

Most cancer support groups find it helpful to develop a few simple ground rules that say how the group will function. Ground rules are created to provide a safe, informal, but structured environment for sharing and learning from each other. People attend support groups for a number of reasons, and simple ground rules will help ensure safety, comfort, and continued focus. Norms and agreements help provide some predictability and stability for returning members and will give new members an idea about how the group works.

It is a good idea to state the agreements at the beginning of each meeting as a reminder and for the benefit of new members.

Suggestions for agreements or ground rules are listed below:

- Our group begins on time and ends on time.
- What we share about our personal lives is confidential and stays in the group.
- We encourage members to share their strengths, skills, successes, and hopes.
- We do not make judgmental comments about other members.
- We listen when someone is talking.
- We avoid interruptions or side conversations.
- We do not discuss people who are not at the meeting.
- Each person has the right to choose to talk or not.
- We each share the responsibility for making the group work.
- The primary responsibility of the leader/facilitator, if there is one, is to ensure that the group is a safe place for members to disclose personal stories.
- When making comments about health care providers or others, members do not use names or identify the individuals and will respect confidentiality.

The Importance of Confidentiality

Since members often interpret the idea of confidentiality in different ways, it is important to define what information your members want to keep confidential. Confidentiality is the practice of keeping private what occurs and is discussed in meetings. Members need to feel safe and comfortable in order to be able to talk openly in groups.

Many groups have an agreement that states that whatever is discussed in the meetings should not be discussed outside of the group. Some groups have a less strict degree of confidentiality that allows

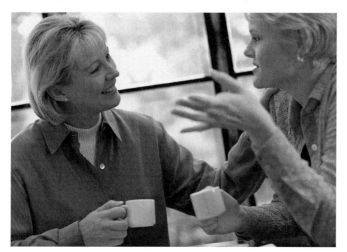

members to talk about the content of the group meetings as long as no identifying information is given. Still other groups use only first names and others have anonymous meetings. In an anonymous meeting, people have the option of not using names. This may be important to some members who are concerned about safeguarding their diagnosis.

> We do not put anybody on our mailing list or send them anything until they give us permission to do so.

Agreements or norms can be drafted by the facilitators when the group is getting started and then shared with all group members. New members might have suggestions for adding to the list if other members feel comfortable with the suggestions. Try to keep the rules simple and easy to remember so that you don't need to write them down. Your group is trying to create intimacy and a welcome place. Don't go overboard with rules and regulations or you will turn people off.

If you have a mailing list for members, decide who will have access to the list. Again, some members may not want to have information about cancer sent to their homes. It is important for the credibility of your group that the membership list be kept confidential and that those entrusted with maintaining the list respect its confidential nature.

The exception to the rule is that confidentiality cannot be maintained in the face of suicidal behaviors. If something like this happens in a group, the members or the facilitators should speak privately to the person making the threats and provide referrals to professional services.

Naming Your Group

Another important step will be choosing a name for your group. This can be a lot of fun for members, and this kind of creativity builds a positive sense of belonging and teamwork. Naming your group and perhaps choosing an image or logo to represent your goals are another way of establishing your identity in your community. When naming a new group or revitalizing an existing group, facilitators need to involve all members. The name and the logo can be used on flyers, newsletters, and other items such as T-shirts to promote the group. For example, a group of adolescents named their group *Lasting Impressions*.[5] This name was chosen to humorously illustrate the impact of chemotherapy, but more importantly to express participants' desire to be remembered and make a contribution, regardless of the length of their lives. The group also designed their own logo, two hands joined and enclosed in two circles, which is on a T-shirt given to each new patient joining the program.

Keeping a Group Record or History

During the hectic start-up period, it helps if you or someone from the organizing group keeps a brief record of decisions and actions. Then, when your group is established, new members can understand what, when, and how decisions were made. Keep contact names and addresses for the people who help. This is a good way to record the history of your group right from the beginning. You might even use this as a story if your group starts to publish a newsletter.

[5] Heiney S, Wells L. *Strategies for Organizing and Maintaining Successful Support Groups. Oncology Nursing Forum* 1989; 16: 803 – 809.

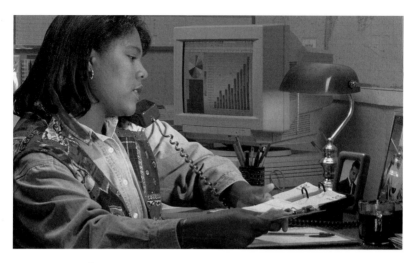

Planning and Publicizing Meetings

Whether you are planning an educational meeting or your first support group meeting, there are some steps you can take to help ensure its success:

- Before planning your own meeting, attend other groups or talk with cancer survivors and patients who have organized similar events.

- Put together a meeting plan or agenda and write it down on a flip chart ahead of time. Post the agenda where everyone can see it and ask if anyone wants to add to it. Then, be ready to change the agenda if the audience wants to add ideas.

- Remember, that the agenda is just a guideline. Don't rush just to cover all of the items. The goal is to generate discussion, not win the agenda race.

- On the day of the meeting, be there early to welcome participants. Your organizing committee should be ready to answer questions, give name tags, and introduce people. Keep the spirit informal, warm, and welcoming. The first impression is important and should reflect warmth and caring for people.

- Have a table set up near the entrance with some refreshments and print materials, brochures, newsletters, or articles you want to share. Ask people to sign in if they want to be contacted by the group after the meeting.

- Arrange the chairs in a circle if possible so that everyone can see one another. Eye contact encourages communication. The flip chart should be located where everyone can easily see it. Leave an opening in the circle for people to join in easily.

- Identify the type of meeting you want and keep the purpose in mind:

  1. To share with others who are living with cancer.

  2. To encourage everyone's ideas about what the group should do.

  3. To set the stage for participation, respect and open communication.

Find a Suitable Meeting Place and Convenient Time

TIME AND PLACE

Consider the people you want to reach when deciding the time and place. For example, the Y-ME National Breast Cancer Organization sponsors lunch-time support groups and education meetings in the downtown business district of Chicago to serve working women. If older breast cancer patients are the people you want to reach, consider daytime meetings along convenient bus routes that are well-lit and in safe areas. If you are choosing a time for the regular support group meeting, keep in mind that it is easier for people to remember the meeting time if it is held in the same place and at the same time, such as the first Monday of each month. Support meetings usually last 1 to 2 hours.

Try to get a free space, such as the local library, church, community center, or social service agency. Avoid the hospital or treatment center if possible; most breast cancer patients and survivors prefer to meet somewhere else. A suitable meeting place will have:

- Safe and free or inexpensive parking;
- Convenient, clean bathrooms;
- Audiovisual equipment; and
- A kitchen.

HOW TO ARRANGE THE ROOM

If you are having a guest speaker or a presentation that uses over-heads, slides, or videos, you need to have people seated in rows (called "theater-style" seating) in order to see the presentation. If you expect a large crowd, seating will also need to be in rows in order to accom-modate and seat the audience comfortably. If you want to have small-group discussions, and people will be asked to write during the meet-ing, small groups seated around tables will work best. If you want to have an informal discussion in a smaller group, have people seated in chairs in a circle or "U" formation to encourage eye contact and create an informal, easy atmosphere.

Finding the perfect room for a meeting can be a challenge, but it is worth the effort. A good meeting place should be:

- Comfortable. If a room is too hot or cold, the chairs are hard or too low, or if there is noise or people wandering through the space, it will be very difficult for people to pay attention, much less share feelings or intimate stories.
- Accessible by wheelchair.
- Near public transit.
- Clean, safe, nonsmoking, and well lit at night.
- Private.
- Large enough to move around without bumping into one another but not too big.
- Available long term.

Before deciding on the room, check on:

- Keys—who is responsible for locking up?
- Room set-up—do you have to arrange the chairs and other things before or after the meeting?
- Availability—what hours can you have the room? Does everyone have to be out at a certain time? What about meetings that go on longer than usual or members who linger and chat?

PUBLICIZE YOUR MEETINGS

Support groups are not always easy to launch, and reaching potential members may take time. Do not forget about your community doctors. They can be an invaluable resource for spreading the word about your meetings.

Free announcements in the community calender sections of the local newspaper, radio, or cable TV can be especially productive. If you are trying to reach underserved populations, try putting notices in the newsletters, cultural centers, grocery stores, schools, and churches that serve the people you want to reach.

Try meeting with the staff at clinics or medical centers that provide care for people from underserved populations and talking with them about your ideas. Talk to community leaders who represent other cultures. Don't be surprised if people are slow to respond to your invitation. It will take time and effort to build new relationships with other communities and cultures.

FLYERS

Use flyers to promote your meeting. Whenever you create a flyer, try to keep the message simple, friendly, and welcoming.

What to include in a flyer:

- *What* is the purpose of the meeting?
- *Who* should come—just women with breast cancer, or family members, friends, and the general public? Is the meeting for women who are newly diagnosed or anyone diagnosed at any time? Can men attend? Can doctors, nurses, or other care providers come?
- *Where* is the meeting? In which room? Give specific and clear directions to the meeting room. A large, simple map is a good idea.
- *When* is the meeting? Give the starting and ending times, and make sure you start and end on time. If you are planning a social time following the event, put that on the flyer. This way, people who are arranging for someone to pick them up won't miss out on anything that is planned.
- *Who* is the contact person, and what is their telephone number? (first names only.)

WHAT TO BRING TO MEETINGS

- Pad of paper or sign-in sheets for names, addresses, and telephone numbers;
- Direction signs to use inside the building, if needed;
- Name tags—reuseable if possible (use first names only);
- Pens;
- Flip chart, paper, and markers; and
- Flyers or brochures.

PLANNING YOUR FIRST ORGANIZATIONAL MEETING

Many breast cancer groups begin with a planning meeting. This is often a meeting with a guest speaker or a facilitator. The purpose of the meeting is to generate interest for your idea and find people who want to join or who want to help the group get going. This first meeting may or may not be a self-help meeting, so you need to be clear with the people you ask to attend. State if this meeting is to talk about starting a new group or if it is the first meeting for group members. This kind of community meeting can serve several purposes:

- Help you to find more interested people;
- Provide information to the general public about the need for cancer groups;
- Help you to find out about other related services;
- Help you to learn what people with cancer in your community want;
- Bring together the people who want to work on cancer issues;
- Generate interest, energy, and enthusiasm; and
- Help to identify possible goals and names.

At the meeting, you will want to ask people to leave their names and addresses if they want to be part of the ongoing group. If the next meeting for the support group has already been planned, hand out flyers stating the date, time, and place.

There are, of course, many details to consider when planning an organizational meeting, such as finding the best location, getting the word out, creating print materials or gathering educational materials, and booking a speaker if you plan to have one. Each member of your organizing group might take on one or two of the tasks.

Planning Your First Support Group Meeting

The first support group meeting will likely include only women living with breast cancer and not the general public. You may find it helpful to refer to the Sample Checklist in this chapter when planning what to do.

The facilitators should begin the meeting by briefly introducing themselves and explaining what the role of the facilitator is. Explain the purpose of the group and suggest some ground rules about confidentiality, speaking one at a time without interruptions, using first names only if that is what your group chooses and no doctors' names or names of health care providers. Then you might begin by asking the participants to talk about what they would like to get from the group and what they would like to give to other members.

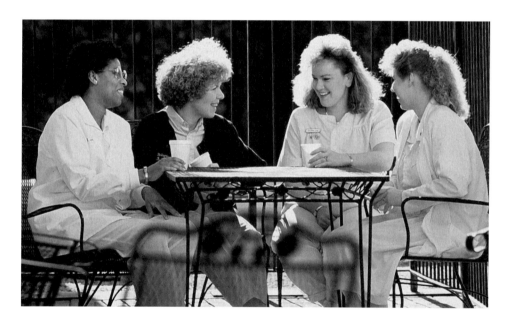

What To Do If You Have A Large Group

If you have a large group (more than 8 to 10), it is wise to break up into smaller groups for discussions. Then, bring the group back together before the close of the meeting. Each smaller group might have a spokesperson who gives a brief summary of the discussion. When the time for the meeting is up, a simple statement of thanks to the people who have come and a reminder of the next meeting time and place is a good ending.

Sample Checklist For Support Group Meetings

- Greet people at the door as they come into the room. Ask them to sign in if they would like to be on the group mailing list.

- Start the meeting on time.

- Welcome everyone and thank them for coming. Try to keep the tone relaxed and friendly. Introduce yourself and the other members of the organizing committee.

- State the purpose of the meeting or show people the agenda if you have one.

- Begin by having a member of the planning group tell her own story and explain how that led to finding others who shared the vision for starting a group.

- At the very first group meeting, go—"round-robin"—meaning that everyone takes a turn speaking—permitting everyone to say what they would like the group to do. Again, discussing the goals and purpose for the group will be important first steps.

- Summarize the discussion and state clearly any actions that will be taken.

- Determine the time and location for future meetings.

- Close the meeting on time. Thank everyone for their contributions. Try to leave time for informal socializing and be available for answering questions following the meeting.

DECIDE HOW OFTEN TO MEET

How often your group should meet depends on the needs of the members and the availability of facilitators. Weekly meetings build familiarity and trust quickly, especially for newly diagnosed patients or these having weekly treatments. For women with a recurrence of cancer, more frequent meetings may help to meet their needs to be with others who understand the urgency of their concerns.

For some mature groups where most of the members know one another, once a month usually works well. But newly diagnosed women may then need to wait several weeks before a group meeting. Often, a telephone support system is arranged to offer peer support from individual members until the group gathers again. Meeting twice a month is one compromise that helps members stay connected and allows new people to join in quickly.

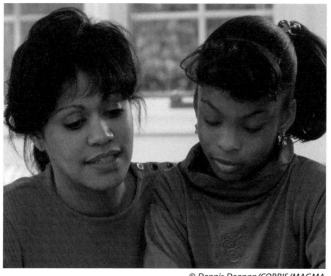

© Dennis Degnan/CORBIS/MAGMA

CHILD CARE

It may be difficult for women with small children to attend meetings. If your group has space and funding, you could arrange to provide child care in another area during the meeting.

Members need to call ahead of the meeting time so that you can plan for the number of children needing care. Make certain that the people providing care are trustworthy, capable, and known to the group, and that they know where the meeting is being held.

TRANSPORTATION

Advertising your meetings well in advance is very helpful to people who have to arrange buses or rides or child care. Members may be able to help one another with driving. The facilitator can raise the question during the business portion of the meeting. Let members know the easiest route to your meeting by public transit.

Final Thoughts

- *Stay in touch with the needs of your members.* From time to time, ask new members about their expectations and needs and what they want from the group. Try to avoid the pitfall of having the core group make all of the decisions and hold the power in the group.

- *Expect your group to experience ups and downs.* Your group will go through changes in attendance and energy. It is natural with all groups and should be expected. Especially when members are struggling during treatments, attendance will depend on individual and group energy.

- Begin by defining your mission, purpose, and goals.

- Establish simple ground rules at the beginning.

- Choose a name and perhaps a logo.

- Arrange a planning or organizational meeting to generate interest.

- Consider the best time, place, and frequency of meetings.

- Plan for issues of transportation and child care.

- Stay in touch with your members' needs and expect some ups and downs.

CHAPTER 4

Facilitation: Leadership from the Heart

> **What you can expect to learn about in this chapter:**
> - Questions for reflecting.
> - Do's and don'ts of facilitation.
> - Qualities or skills to look for when choosing a facilitator.
> - Creating an effective group environment.
> - Different types of facilitation.
> - Recognizing when a facilitator is doing too much.
> - Preventing facilitator burnout.

Leadership is not domination but the art of
persuading people to work toward a common goal.

DANIEL GOLEMAN, EMOTIONAL INTELLIGENCE[6]

Group facilitation in the self-help model has been referred to as "leadership from behind" or "servant leadership." It is an approach to facilitation that is preferred to more aggressive or sophisticated interventions.

When we are asked to lead a team or a group, it is often because we have special professional skills or experiences or a position of authority that is different and valued more than other members of the group. In a self-help group, the facilitator is a group member with a specific role to play to encourage members to participate in discussions. Usually, facilitators of support groups are chosen because they are good role models for others and because they demonstrate genuine compassion, caring and warmth. Often, our ability to facilitate a group effectively, comes from the insights that we have gained through our own struggles with breast cancer, combined with an awareness of how to encourage others.

---

[6] Goleman D. *Emotional Intelligence*. New York, NY: Bantam Books, 1995.

Understanding Your Interest in Leadership

It may be helpful to begin by reflecting on what you have learned as a cancer survivor. The following questions may be helpful in remembering what your initial reactions were, how your relationships were affected, and how others helped:

Ask yourself:

- What did I think about people who had cancer before I was diagnosed?
- How did I feel when I first heard the diagnosis?
- Was it different from what I expected or wanted?
- What would I write to someone with a similar diagnosis?
- What was the hardest part of the diagnosis?
- Who was the easiest person to talk to?
- Was I angry with the doctor? Why?
- What did I do about being angry?
- How do I feel about the help I got from doctors and nurses?
- How have people reacted?
- How did I deal with my fear or loneliness?
- What problems have I overcome?
- What problems am I still struggling with?
- What were my goals or dreams before the diagnosis?
- What are my dreams now?
- How has my life changed?
- If I have learned anything special about life because of my situation, it is _____.

You might also consider what it is that you have to offer other breast cancer patients and survivors. Which of these suggestions fits for you?

- I want to share my experience with others.
- I want to return the kindness I have had from others.
- I want to be involved in something important.
- It helps me to know that I am not alone.
- My cancer has been treated and I am well. Now I want to give back.
- I am grateful for my health and want to tell others about the things that helped.
- I believe that support groups can help cancer patients to heal.
- Helping other people helps me.

Thinking back to the time of your own diagnosis and remembering what helped you through the difficult time of treatment may guide you through the first meetings of your group when you hear other women starting on their journey.

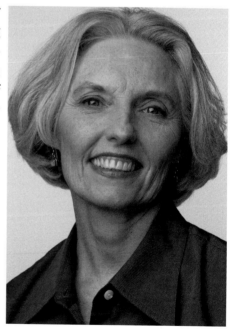

Understanding the Difference between *Leading* and *Facilitating*

The leader of self-help groups does not direct the group in the traditional manner of a group leader. Rather, the leader guides the members during their discussion. The facilitator is not controlling or directing but is attentive to the needs of the group and responsive to maintaining a safe, compassionate atmosphere.

The job of facilitating is a little bit like being a guide on a river raft: the guide coaches everyone involved and helps steer through rough water but doesn't do all of the work. Like a river-raft guide, the facilitators guide others, maintaining balance, searching for the safe passage. At times, the facilitators might not appear to be working at all, but because they have a watchful eye on how members are reacting, they can anticipate what may be up ahead. They can bring attention to where the group is at, alert members to issues, and suggest ways to get through the rough spots!

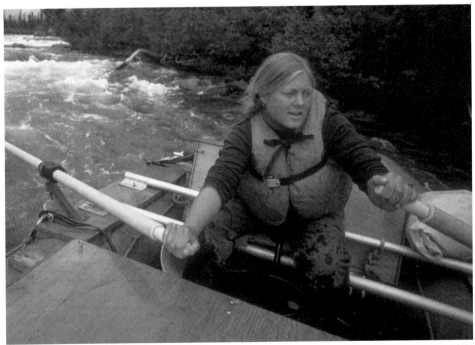

© Joel W. Rogers/CORBIS/MAGMA

The following is a list of some of the "Do's" and "Don'ts" for facilitators:

DO'S	DON'TS
• Encourage members to explore answers	• Assume that you need to have all of the answers
• Participate	• Take over
• Provide information	• Lecture
• Encourage everyone to speak	• Pressure or obligate members to talk
• Empathize	• Focus on yourself
• Clarify members' feelings	• Prevent others in the group from helping to clarify someone's feelings
• Let members explore feelings	• Rescue them
• Protect members from hostility	• Block expressions of anger
• Support and balance different views	• Take sides
• Prepare an agenda	• Insist on sticking to the agenda
• Use structure and predictability to reduce anxiety	• Substitute structure for control
• Acknowledge group tensions	• Avoid tough issues
• Use humor to reduce stress or bring members together	• Use humor to distract or avoid difficult issues

Choosing a Facilitator

Many effective groups are led by women who have a natural talent for making a group feel warm and welcoming. These women will often have a great deal of common sense, good hearts, and lots of energy and courage. You might begin to notice them because they are good listeners and other people seem to be drawn to them. When you are searching for a facilitator, the following talents may be helpful. Look for someone who:

- Understands the difference between a self-help support group and a therapy group.
- Is prepared to promote an atmosphere of acceptance and understanding.
- Is able to facilitate the development of trusting relationships.

- Is a good listener.
- Has a positive attitude toward their own adjustment and is able to be objective.
- Has training or demonstrated ability to facilitate groups.
- Is willing to continue to learn, help with evaluations, and accept feedback. [7]

Facilitators can draw upon these past experiences, training, and common sense to know when it is time to intervene and when it is time to be silent.

> I think one of the most difficult things is really knowing when to come in. When is the point that you say, "Sue, I know this is important for you, but we are really going to have to move on with someone else now...." Interrupting someone or just getting them to wrap it up—that is really hard.

Effective Facilitation

Evaluations[8] from successful cancer support groups have described some of the characteristics of effective facilitators. These characteristics include being:

- Caring,
- Involved,
- Sensitive,
- Understanding,
- Accepting,
- Aware,
- Confident,
- Active, and
- Fair.

[7] From *Guidelines on Support and Self-Help Groups*. American Cancer Society, 1994. Used with permission.

[8] Cella DF, Sarafian B, Snider PR, Yellen SB, Winicour P. Evaluation of a community-based cancer support group. *Journal of Psycho-Oncology*, 1993;2:123 – 132.

Effective facilitators understand the key needs of group members. As we have said before, all groups are different, and there is no one right way to go about starting or managing a group. An effective group facilitator understands the key needs of members, helps to maintain self-esteem and open communication and works to build mutual trust.

Effective facilitators understand why members come and go, without making judgements. Members often start attending a group when they are newly diagnosed, then continue until the end of treatment. Once treatment ends, many women decide that it is time to move on and will leave the group, knowing that they can return anytime.

Some women choose to stay involved with the group in a different way through volunteering and giving back to other women. Each member chooses what is right for them, according to their needs and abilities. Again, the spirit of self-help is that we take what we need, give what we can, and appreciate others, without judgment.

Effective facilitators help create a safe, welcoming environment. The facilitator can encourage the development of a safe group climate by:

- Helping members to accept and appreciate each others differences,

- Respecting members' right to limit how much they want to share or reveal, and

- Using humor to balance intensity.

Group facilitators help support to happen through education and encouraging problem solving by group members. The facilitator models compassionate behaviors and members reinforce the positive and productive behaviors that promote self-esteem. The supportive group environment may at times become tense, but the facilitator knows how to prevent or reduce tension by providing a structure that gives the group direction and support and by planning for laughter and fun to balance the seriousness.

Meetings need to have a balance of providing education and learning along with support; otherwise, members may keep coming back, but they socialize and share friendships rather than being focused on learning or coping with cancer. If this happens in your group, it is time to re-examine or evaluate the groups' purpose by inviting members to discuss how to focus on breast cancer support.

TIPS

✓ *You should talk about the role of the facilitators at the beginning of each meeting for the sake of any new people. This will help everyone to understand what their own role is and that the members all share responsibility for the success of the group.*

✓ *Remember that the best facilitators are the ones who make other people feel welcome and comfortable. You might not hear them talking during the group meeting but their presence helps all of the other members to do their work.*

Types of Facilitation

ROTATING FACILITATION

One way to ensure that the leadership is shared in a cancer group is to rotate the job of facilitator. This allows all of the members who have the skills and desire to share in the responsibility of managing the work of the group and gaining different perspectives on what the job requires. Plan ahead and schedule in advance who will facilitate each meeting. Remember to be flexible. The facilitators are group members and their health and other commitments may change and you will need to have a back-up plan in place. With rotating facilitation, another person should be prepared to take over if the member who was scheduled is not available.

SHARED OR CO-FACILITATION

Shared facilitation or co-facilitation means that two or more people take on the facilitation tasks and roles. It is very popular with groups that decide to keep the same facilitators for a long period of time.

There are many benefits of using shared facilitation:

- Different members have different strengths and skills and can be used to balance the tasks of content and process (discussed in the next chapter).
- Co-facilitators can learn from one another.
- Having someone to debrief with after meetings helps the facilitator to prevent burnout.
- Co-facilitators can lean on one another when the going gets rough or when they are stuck.
- It is easier to stay focused and on time.
- The emotional burden of time and energy is shared.
- Co-facilitators can provide encouragement and support for each other.

When a Facilitator Is Doing Too Much

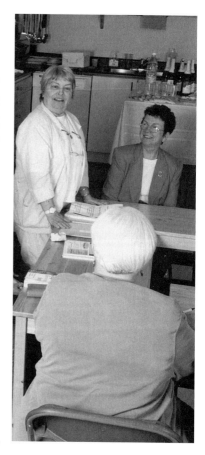

When all eyes are focused on the facilitators much of the time, or when the facilitators are doing most of the talking and answering all of the questions, the facilitators are doing too much. Again, the role of the facilitator is to make the work of the group *easy*, not *to do* the work of the group. Members have to be involved and responsible for what happens in the meetings or the group will not work. Members will always look to the facilitators to answer questions and solve problems, and they will not have the experience of solving the problems for themselves. These steps may be helpful in preventing the facilitators from becoming overinvolved:

- The facilitators should keep opening remarks welcoming, brief, and on topic.
- The facilitators should not respond right away, even when questioned directly.
- Make sure others have a chance to respond first. If support is needed, members may take a moment before offering it.
- When no members are responding to questions, try to draw members in by using open-ended questions such as "Has anyone had any experience with the problem?"

Preventing Facilitator Burnout

Burnout is a serious problem with no easy solutions. However, you can work to organize your group so that no one is unduly stressed. A few suggestions for preventing burnout include:

- Have more than one or two facilitators and rotate the job.
- Limit the length of time people are expected to serve. Imagining that your job as facilitator will never end can cause burnout.
- Develop structured guidelines. Some groups develop specific guidelines on how to handle difficult situations or problem behavior. This policy can relieve the facilitator from worrying too much about how they might handle situations. Written guidelines help ensure continuity and consistency between contact persons and can serve as a guide for new facilitators.
- Write down your feelings and comments in the group record or journal you keep for your group. Debrief with your co-facilitator after meetings as a way of giving and getting feedback and support for your efforts.

- Find a helping professional in your community and develop a helping or mentoring relationship. Professionals can be a valuable resource for facilitators and can help with problem solving, referrals, and other support.

- Make a plan for bringing in new group members and preparing them to do facilitation. Plan to register them for training or skills workshops that might help.

- Coach the new facilitator and ease your way out.

- Share with your group when you start to feel overburdened. You too are a member, and sharing with other members, is what it is all about.

Keeping A Group Record, History, or Journal

No matter which kind of facilitation your group decides to use, it is helpful to keep a history or a brief record of meetings. The information that is recorded should not identify members and should respect confidentiality and any other norms and agreements of the group. This record is an important history of your group's activities and decisions and will be very helpful to new facilitators. Record decisions made, ground rules or agreements, special guests or speakers, and any significant discussions. Quotation can also be important but, again, respect confidentiality. Let the group members know that a brief record is kept and that they are welcome to read the notes at any time.

KEY MESSAGES FROM THIS CHAPTER:

- Understand the needs of the group's members.

- Trust the process and share facilitation.

- Encourage a warm, welcoming group environment.

- Pay attention to the ground rules.

- Inspire others.

- Keep a record or history.

CHAPTER 5

Group Tasks and Skills

What you can expect to learn about in this chapter:
- The difference between content of discussions and group process.
- How to encourage open discussion and share time.
- How to use silence appropriately.

Facilitators and members share the following tasks:

- Starting and ending the meeting on time.

- Setting the agenda.

- Keeping the discussion on topic.

- Setting guidelines or agreements and reminding members when appropriate.

- Suggesting a periodic review or evaluation.

- Keeping a record about meetings.

- Modeling compassion and supportive behavior.

- Sharing information.

Developing good group skills takes a lot of time and practice. Don't be discouraged if there are problems. Mistakes happen. People with cancer share very strong emotions and group meetings can be rocky. Staying open to learning from mistakes helps the group maintain safety and trust. Practice forgiveness and good humor with yourself and with members of your group. Talk to other facilitators and breast cancer group leaders or helping professionals. Ask for their ideas or suggestions and problem solve together. Share what you learn with the other members of your group. They, too, want the group to work well. There are a number of skills described in this chapter that members can practice to ensure that meetings work for everyone.

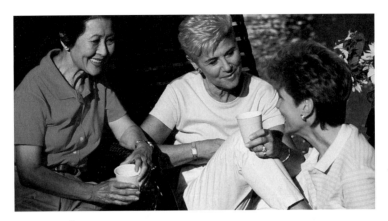

Content and Process

Facilitators will need to keep track of what the group is discussing (content) and the way (process) in which the members are interacting with each other. Again, having two group members who act as co-facilitators will help to ensure that both the content and the process are being attended to. The facilitator can help with content by answering questions or suggesting where to find information or resources.

Some of us will be more comfortable with sitting back and listening and watching the way in which each member is reacting and contributing. Others may have identified personal skills that will help with the subject being discussed. You will need to draw upon your experiences in groups to know where your particular skills are and to apply them in your role as facilitator and group member. Again, you might find it helpful to refer to the Personal Skills Inventory (Appendix A) for some of the skills that you can apply to facilitating self-help groups.

Effective group process can help members:

- Identify the common ways members experience cancer,
- Be aware of the sense of release that happens after emotions are expressed,
- Give and receive support and help,
- Share information,
- Find hope,
- Be aware of how others cope,
- Foster group trust and bonding, and
- Develop a common purpose and meaning.

The process of keeping the group focused and working effectively is challenging. When members become overwhelmed with negative emotions or one member seems to be taking over the group time, using suggestions from the list on page 62 can help to bring the group back to a positive focus. This does not mean that a cancer support group should never talk about negative or sad issues; rather, we suggest finding a way to bring the members through the discussion in order to be able to end on a positive note. Cancer support groups cannot take away the pain or suffering of a cancer diagnosis; groups can help members to learn to cope and adjust to life after a diagnosis of cancer.

For example, the facilitator can ask questions such as *"I'm feeling really sad about Mary's death and I'm wondering if others are feeling the same way? Would someone else like to talk about how they are feeling right now?"* The question helps to guide the group in exploring feelings that might otherwise never be voiced. In this way, the facilitator shares something intimate about herself that models for other members what they might try. The ultimate goal is to discover that sharing and caring does ease the pain of loneliness and fear and that coping is possible even in the face of sadness or death.

Empathizing, Not Sympathizing

Empathizing is not saying "I know how you feel." It is trying to understand another cancer survivor's experience in the way she has described it. Allow the speaker time to fully express herself. Allow her to become aware of her feelings and to begin dealing with them. Be present with your body, mind, and heart and try to resist the temptation to offer your own solutions and thoughts.

Being sympathetic means feeling sorry for someone. When we offer sympathy, we are not on an equal footing with the person we are listening to or helping. Our feelings of pity will be obvious. This response will not likely be helpful and, in the long term, some people may regret having shared intimate and vulnerable emotions with you.

Using Group Silence

Many of us are not comfortable with silence and feel the need to fill the void. Silence can be a very useful tool when used with skill and awareness. Silence can allow group members to gather their thoughts and help to slow down the discussion. It can have a calming influence for members who may have become frightened or whose thoughts are scattered.

A prolonged silence, however, can create negative feelings, and members may wonder if there is a problem. Timing is important here, but generally the facilitator should respect the silence and allow members to resume the conversation when they are ready.

Asking Open-Ended Questions

Open-ended questions such as *"Can you talk about how you might like the group to be helpful with this problem?"* require the person speaking to expand on her idea or comment. Open-ended questions invite the person talking to continue the discussion and explore difficult or complex issues knowing that there is a willing listener who is interested in and committed to hearing from her.

A closed-ended question such as *"Can we talk about this at the break?"* can be answered with a simple yes or no and may be helpful if you need to stop someone from talking too long. Try to limit the use of open-ended questions when you are coming to the end of the meeting time.

Try to discourage asking why questions. Those questions can sound judgmental or blaming. For example, *"Why did you go to that doctor?"* may sound like the patient is responsible for getting poor treatment.

Sharing Experiences and Strengths

When someone tells you her story, you can show that you have listened by affirming the messages she has conveyed. You can say *"It sounds as if that conversation with your daughter was really important for you"* or *"It took courage to say what was in your heart."* Even when stories are hard to talk about, you can affirm the strengths that people have shown.

By sharing common experiences, your group will develop a cohesive and intimate group spirit. It can be comforting to learn that other cancer survivors have had to face similar experiences and some of the same feelings, and that they have found ways to cope.

Active Listening

> The most valuable gift we can give
> another person is the quality of our attention.

Dr. Richard Moss [9]

Becoming an active listener is a learned skill that is taught by many volunteer or social service organizations. This is a skill that cancer group members will find they need to use frequently, and one that is useful in all of our relationships. Consider investing time in getting this training and encourage other group facilitators to become trained. Ask your local nonprofit organizations and social service agencies who train volunteers if they offer programs in active listening.

Active listening [10] is a way of communicating that helps clarify another person's way of thinking. Most of us are in the habit of listening to others, but active listen-ing is more than just hearing words. Active listening involves using skills that enable the listener to understand meaning. It means paying attention to the speaker's use of specific words, the meaning of the words used, and the feelings and actions that go along with the words.

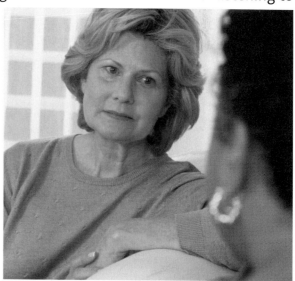

---

[9] Moss R. *The Second Miracle*. Berkeley, CA: Celestial Arts Publishing, 1995.

[10] Adapted from *Section 2, Listening Skills-ME Hotline Training Program*.
  Y-ME National Breast Cancer Organization: Chicago, IL, 1995.

Women diagnosed with breast cancer often feel very threatened and defensive. They may feel like they have lost control of their life and their self-image is weakened. Active listening allows the person talking to explore her self-image knowing that the listener fully accepts her as she is without reservation or expectation. Active listening promotes personal growth and the strengthening of a person's sense of self. The good listener provides:

- Noncritical acceptance,
- A genuine sense of equality and freedom to speak, and
- Understanding and warmth.

You might also find it helpful to pay attention to the responses that stop people from talking:

- Changing the subject;
- Not making eye contact;
- Being easily distracted—answering the telephone, reading;
- Questioning decisions or making judgments;
- Giving advice or offering opinions;
- Asking the speaker to constantly repeat what they are saying;
- Interrupting;
- Showing pity;
- Being glib or philosophical; and
- Rushing the speaker.

Active listening involves behaviors and attitudes. An easy way to remember them is the formula **BRIEF**:

B Body posture including movements and gestures that communicate awareness.

R Respect for the other person's right to speak and be heard.

I Intimacy, which involves the creation of a safe, caring environment in which ideas and feelings can be freely expressed without fear of judgment.

E Eye contact communicates interest and attention.

F Following, which is both verbal and nonverbal. Verbal following includes the use of open-ended questions and minimal words. Nonverbal following includes nodding, smiling, and appropriate facial gestures.

KEY MESSAGES FROM THIS CHAPTER:

- Keep track of content and process during discussions.

- Empathize, don't sympathize.

- Help new people connect with others in the group.

- Practice and model active listening skills.

CHAPTER 6

Managing Difficult Behaviors and Other Challenges

> **What you can expect to learn about in this chapter:**
> • How cancer affects self-esteem.
> • Recognizing and managing problem behaviors.
> • Dealing with angry members.

Like most groups, cancer self-help groups will face challenges. Members can learn how to become effective at confronting difficult behaviors, without offending. By learning and practicing these skills, members will become less dependent on the facilitator to handle issues. Members will also improve their own sense of self-esteem and competency when they are more in control of problem situations.

Self-Esteem and Cancer[11]

> Ninety percent of what we do is listening and sharing and making women feel good about themselves, and getting through it and coming out the other end of the tunnel even better than before.

We have included this section on self-esteem to help your group members understand that the group can have a powerful effect on members self-esteem—both positively or negatively. When self-esteem is threatened by illness, our behaviors, as a result, can be difficult or challenging for other people. We don't necessarily want to be threatening or frightening to others—especially people who might be able to help—but illness can cause us to be very defensive and not act our best. Understanding how cancer affects self-esteem may provide some insights about how to help yourself and others.

---

[11] Courtesy of Hugh Huntington, The Huntington Group, Asheville, NC.

Self-esteem is a measure of how you feel about who you are and how much you enjoy being who you are. People with high self-esteem don't always feel good about what is happening to them—such as a diagnosis of cancer—and they might want to change their circumstances. But they do not want to become someone else. Positive or high self-esteem is a good foundation for mental and emotional health. If you go through life with low self-esteem, you will always feel like something is wrong or missing in your life. Because you live with yourself all of the time, it is important that you enjoy your own company or you will always be looking for something or someone else to make you happy.

Self-esteem is a fluid or dynamic quality that changes constantly. When your life changes for the better or for the worse, your self-esteem moves up or down. Like a bucket full of water, when your self-esteem is high, you can dip in and draw from the bucket without feeling that you have lost anything. If you have lived with low self-esteem for a long time, another drop out of the bucket can leave us feeling completely empty. Understandably, the effects of cancer and its treatments can have a powerful effect on self-esteem. There are many sources of self-esteem; we will discuss four.

RECOGNITION

The first source of self-esteem is recognition or being valued and cared about, particularly by those who know and love us. Recognition is a simple process, but when we go without it, our self esteem drops. Recognition can be a warm hello or a hug from a family member. It can also come from our boss asking how we feel. But when we have cancer and are in treatment, the change in daily routine means that we often don't see the people who give us recognition. If they are care givers or family members we live with, they see us so much that they forget to acknowledge us.

ACHIEVEMENT

The second source of self-esteem is achievement, accomplishment, or mastery. Long-term accomplishments often have to do with major goals such as getting married, raising kids, building a business, being promoted, going to school, and staying in good physical shape. Short-

Living with Breast Cancer

term accomplishments such as keeping the house clean, mowing the lawn, preparing a meal, and participating in sports or family activities are usually achieved more often. Of course, cancer and cancer treatments can leave us feeling sick or exhausted and unable to do these things. Again, not being able to benefit from the usual sense of accomplishment will affect our self-esteem.

POWER AND INFLUENCE

The third source of self-esteem is referred to as power, control, and influence over our lives and the way we lead them. Having power means having the ability to make choices and make things happen the way we want them to happen. Having cancer and needing to take treatments will mean having to make clinic appointments and spend time in hospitals or treatment centers. Cancer can interfere with travel plans, weddings, planning a family, school, and careers. We lose the ability to control how we spend our time, at least temporarily. Of the four sources of self-esteem, power and influence seem to carry the greatest weight; it can take us down and build us up faster than the other sources.

PERSONAL VALUES AND BELIEFS

The last source of self-esteem is the ability to behave in ways that match our personal values and beliefs. These values and beliefs are unique to each person. A value is often based on a belief or a combination of beliefs. Personal values and beliefs can come from various sources such as spirituality or religion, family, work, education, relationships, sports activities or fitness, art, music, and personal appearance. Our ability to live and act on these values helps us to maintain our self-esteem. If religious belief is considered valuable, being able to attend services or prayers will be an important way to maintain self-esteem, especially during a diagnosis of cancer. Being unable to play music, create arts and crafts, practice sports, or participate in a regular exercise program will have an impact on self-esteem for people who value these activities.

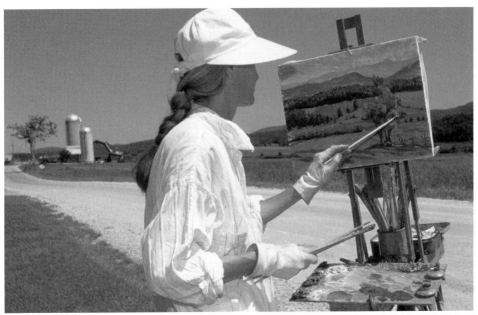

How a Self-Help Group Affects Members' Self-Esteem

If a group member is missing the recognition she received from significant people in her life or is feeling uncared for, other group members can encourage her to recognize and ask for what she needs. To help foster a sense of achievement or accomplishment, group members can encourage one another to take on small tasks. Even small accomplishments will increase self-esteem and stop the downward spiral of negative thinking. Group members recognize the significance of these efforts and can share and celebrate the small milestones toward well-being.

Assisting people in finding out about treatment options is an excellent way to regain a sense of power and influence. Helping them prepare a list of questions or guiding them through the confusion of the cancer clinic can renew someone's self-confidence immeasurably.

You can also help someone get back into the routine she valued before diagnosis. By doing so, you help the person to regain her personal values and beliefs. Being able to once again do simple tasks such as wearing make-up, managing personal hygiene, preparing a meal, walking or other moderate exercise, going to church, and listening to music helps to increase self-esteem. The basic guideline is to help someone to find her way back to doing the things she valued by encouraging her to explore possibilities.

Finally, for some people, being a cancer patient can become a source of power and increase self-esteem. After all, cancer can seem very helpful: you get the support and sympathy from family and friends, you get time off from work and other duties, or you get special recognition. These are sometimes referred to as the "secondary gains of illness." Problems develop when you dwell on or become attached to suffering and illness as a way of avoiding change.

We should not confuse having cancer with being worthy of love and attention. Being worthy of the love and attention of others has to do with being and acting in loving ways and appreciating others. Otherwise, we might be tempted to use our cancer experience to exploit the goodwill of others. The best advice here is to nurture good relationships—both when we are sick and when we are well.

Common Challenges in Breast Cancer Groups: Managing Problem Behaviors

At some time, every group will have someone whose behavior causes problems for other members. Here are some of the most common problem behaviors and suggestions for how to handle the situations, in a constructive way and without offending.[12]

THE MONOPOLIZER

This person needs to tell her story at every meeting in every discussion and wants all of the group time and attention.

What to try. Acknowledge and redirect her energy. If she is new to the group or newly diagnosed, she may be very needy of your group's attention. Do not allow the behavior to continue. Explain to her the guidelines and agreements that help members to be respectful and share time. For the benefit of the group, it may eventually become necessary to confront this person and tell her that she cannot contin-

---

[12] *Identifying and Handling Problem Behaviors: Guidelines on Support and Self-Help Groups.* American Cancer Society, 1994:63. Adapted with permission.

ue to monopolize the group. Give her the choice of continuing with the group and respecting the agreements and the needs of other members. As a last resort, when all else fails, privately ask the person to leave the group.

THE HELP-REJECTING COMPLAINER

This person complains all of the time but refuses any helpful suggestions. She uses expressions like "yes, but" a lot.

What to try. Group members can confront the complainer and build on the positive experiences that everyone in the group shares. Focus on things that can be done. Ask specifically what the complainer was hoping to get from the group and ask her to focus on how she and the other group members can problem solve together.

THE HOSTILE MEMBER

Unlike people who use anger to move into constructive action, the hostile member directs anger at other members of the group. This kind of person may also be very hostile outside the group as well.

What to try. Actively protect the safety of the group by setting firm limits: respect, no interruptions, no judgments. Ask the hostile member if she understands the group agreements and norms. If the person will not or cannot conform to the group rules, the facilitator should privately ask her to leave.

THE WITHDRAWN MEMBER

This person rarely or never talks or participates in the group.

What to try. Encourage her participation. Watch her body language carefully and try calling on her when you notice that she is responding, when her eyes light up during a certain discussion, or if she nods when someone else is talking. At the beginning or end of the meeting, use check-in times during which everyone says a few words to help them link with the rest of the group. Support and encourage everyone's participation but do not demand it. Good listeners, as discussed in the previous chapter, are as valuable to a group as those members who speak regularly.

THE MENTAL HEALTH PROBLEM MEMBER

This member is suicidal, psychotic, or deeply depressed and does not do well in support groups.

What to try. If the condition is obviously a problem, refer the person to mental health services or groups. Let her know that group participation may be appropriate when she is able to cope. Remember, that there is a clear difference between self-help and mental health services or therapy. Some people will need help that is beyond your group's ability and you would do them and yourself a disservice if you did not refer them to the appropriate help.

SUMMARY

These behaviors will threaten the spirit and effectiveness of the group. When the facilitator or other members confront the problem behavior and set limits, they help bring the group back to being effective, safe, and welcoming. When you must ask someone to leave the group, let her know that she is welcome to return when she is able and willing to respect the agreements.

Other Challenges

THE ANGRY MEMBER

Cancer group members acknowledge that many women need to vent anger, which is often related to delays in diagnosis or a perceived physician insensitivity in communicating diagnosis, treatment, or likelihood of cure. Although the story of a group member's experience is always welcomed and supported no matter how angry she is, it is also made clear that it is unacceptable to identify doctors.

There also seems to be a collective understanding in cancer self-help groups that staying stuck in this anger is counterproductive. Expressing anger is usually the first step in taking responsibility for one's health care and using the group in a supportive, constructive way in order to begin to heal and learn to cope.

- Cancer affects self-esteem.

- All members are responsible for helping the group work.

- Learn to limit problem behavior by sticking with the group guidelines.

Chapter 7

Assertive Caring

What you can expect to learn about in this chapter:
- What is assertive caring.
- How and when to use assertive caring.
- Different approaches to decision making.

In the <u>Self-Help Leader's Handbook: Leading Effective Meetings</u>,[13] the authors describe assertive caring as a way to say no without offending. Assertive caring is used to deal with disruptive behaviors and allows all members to benefit from the group.

The four steps in assertive caring are:

1. Provide a statement of understanding.

2. Set limits.

3. Suggest an alternative and check for agreement.

How to Use Assertive Caring

1. Provide a Statement of Understanding

The first part of assertive caring consists of making a statement of understanding. For example, if a group member is taking up a great deal of time with the same problems at each meeting, you might say *"I understand you are having trouble getting help from your husband and family since your diagnosis."*

---

[13] *Self-Help Leader's Handbook: Leading Effective Meetings.* The Research and Training Center on Independent Living, University of Kansas:, Lawrence, KS, 1991.

2. Set Limits

The second part of assertive caring is setting limits. Setting limits involves letting the person know why you need to change the situation. For example, saying *"Many of us have struggled with our families' reactions. I know I did. We have spent time exploring options with you. But right now, we need to let other people have a chance to talk."* Saying this to the person lets her become aware that she has taken up too much group time on a particular topic and that she must respect the needs of the other members.

3. Suggest an Alternative and Check for Agreement

The final part of assertive caring involves suggesting an alternative and making sure that the arrangement suggested is okay with all of the members—for example, *"Perhaps you could continue talking about this after the meeting. Would that work for you?"*

Of course, assertive caring won't work in every challenging situation. If the situation is more complicated, the whole group may want to brainstorm alternatives. It is important to be flexible, to be caring, and to find solutions that don't embarrass or disrespect the group member.

When to Use Assertive Caring

- When one member of the group talks too much.
- When frequent interruptions with irrelevant and/or inappropriate talk are made by one member.
- When a member of the group frequently responds with "yes, but" for suggestions by other group members.
- When a member repeatedly brings up issues not related to breast cancer.
- When a member consistently arrives late and/or interrupts group meetings.
- When a member appears to need more help or different help than the group can give.
- When a member makes discriminatory or offensive remarks.

Making Group Decisions

Important decisions, made by one person, don't happen very often in self-help groups. This is because self-help groups place a high value on the involvement of members in all matters that affect the group. Keeping the administrative needs of your group simple will limit the kinds of decision-making problems that you face.

MAJORITY RULES

This is the most common method of group decision making. Issues are discussed, and as long as more than half of the members agree to the same alternative, the decision is made. This way of coming to a decision can be useful on issues where consensus (when everyone agrees) will not work. A dissatisfied minority, however, will remain. The majority rules method is useful when there is little time for making a decision, and it can be effective when the decision made is not a critical one.

CONSENSUS

Most self-help groups strive to attain consensus when making decisions that are important to the whole group. When deciding on such things as the purpose of the group, the kinds of members, and when and where to meet, everyone should have a chance or feel that they have had a chance in influencing the final decision. Consensus can only work in groups in which the members basically like and trust one another. Otherwise, differences of opinion will not be valued and will be seen as threatening. The advantage of a decision made by consensus is that

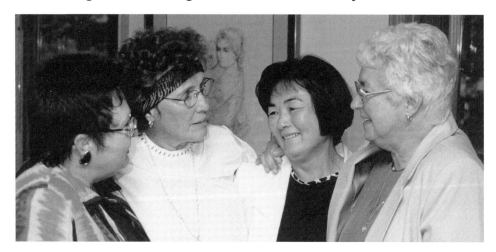

practically all members will be committed to it. Many groups aim for "modified consensus." In this model, most of the group is in agreement, and those who disagree may go along with the rest of the group after their opinions have been heard.

It can take a lot of time and energy to achieve consensus: everyone needs to be heard. As well, consensus rarely occurs since there will always be at least as many points of view as there are members. But, for the important decisions, attempting to reach consensus is very useful. The process brings group members together and ensures greater commitment to carry through on the decisions.

KEY MESSAGES FROM THIS CHAPTER:

- Assertive caring is a way of saying no without offending.
- Using assertive caring helps minimize disruptive behaviors and allows all group members to benefit from the group.
- Group decisions should be arrived at using majority rule (for less important decisions) or by consensus (more important decisions).

CHAPTER 8

Managing Challenges and Changes from Grief and Loss

> **What you can expect to learn about in this chapter:**
> • Understanding the process of grief.
> • Understanding how groups can be helpful in coping with grief and loss.

Loss and grief are part of breast cancer groups. However much we want to maintain a positive and optimistic approach to support groups, the reality is that we must also be prepared when members talk about their fear of dying, the losses some women experience with mastectomy and lumpectomy, the recurrence of disease, and the deaths of members. If groups ignore this reality, then they are unlikely to be able to meet members' needs.

It takes a lot of courage to face fears about our own death and dying. Women go to breast cancer groups and find other "veteran" cancer survivors who share their experience, strength, and hope.

But the groups will also include other members whose disease gets worse and not better. There will be deaths among group members. The effects of these deaths on group members can be devastating, especially when members have also become friends.

Breast cancer support group members face a huge dilemma. On the one hand is the desire to maintain a hopeful attitude and not overwhelm new members with stories of loss and grief. On the other hand is the desire to extend support to members who are dying and to grieve for the friends who have died. Often, cancer self-help groups that are unable to meet the needs of seriously ill people have to deal with anger, both from the person who is ill and from other members who want to be more helpful.

I don't think they always supported her. I feel like they didn't want to hear it ....the few times that death got brought up at the meeting were the times that people didn't come back. And that made me angry, but again, now I'm accepting and realizing maybe they just couldn't.

By now you might be thinking that starting or joining a cancer support group is not such a good idea. Maybe you are thinking that it will be too painful or remind you too much of your own fear of death. This is especially true if, like most cancer survivors, you are struggling with your own grief over the loss of your good health, sexuality, or femininity. Perhaps, like many, you would prefer to just maintain a positive attitude and stay away from people who are really ill or maybe even dying. After all, most people want to put cancer behind them and go on with their lives. This is the right choice for many people; only you can decide what is right for you.

However, if you choose to join a breast cancer support group or start a new one, you will also have an opportunity to be with people through some of the most difficult and rewarding days of their lives. This chapter is about preparing and understanding how a breast cancer group can be helpful to those members whose cancer is getting worse and whose lives are ending and for the members who are trying to be supportive. However, the greatest teachers for this work will be the members of your group who struggle with this challenge.

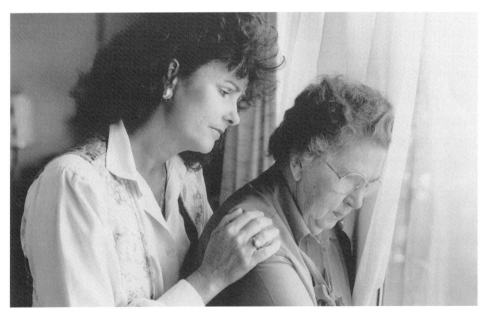

Living with Breast Cancer

If you are struggling with a dying member right now and your group is feeling overwhelmed, help is probably available in your community. Churches and funeral homes often have staff who are trained in bereavement counseling. Hospices and groups for bereaved families have people who are experienced in dealing with death and dying and may have someone who can meet with your group. The right person can become an ongoing resource to discuss with members how to be helpful, how to cope with projections about their own death, and how to use ceremonies that can help remember and celebrate the life lost.

Again, there is no easy way to do this and there is no right or wrong way. But having an understanding of the process of grief and healing can be helpful for facilitators and other group members.

Managing Grief and Change in Cancer Support Groups

Grief is a highly personal and normal response to a life-changing event and a process that can lead to healing and personal growth. Grief is the process that helps us to adapt to the changes that come with loss. Grief helps us to create our story about the lost relationship. Grief is like an intimate record of our emotional, physical, spiritual, and social relationship with the person or thing that has been lost.

The process of grief takes time—often a lot more time than we think. It touches everything about our life and is very hard work. It takes physical and emotional energy to cope with the changes that come with grief. It can be painful and may sometimes seem neverending. The following are some things that other breast cancer groups have done that helped with grief:

- Having other members share their stories and memories of the person.

- Having the facilitator initiate a discussion about the woman who died by asking "Is there anything you would like to say about her?"

- Sitting close together in the circle.

- One member asking for a hug and getting surrounded by 12 members.
- Reflecting for a moment in silence.
- Laughing and celebrating the joy of having known a beautiful woman.
- Lighting a candle and watching in silence as the flame danced and glowed.
- Making a card together for her family.

Groups can help provide the support necessary during, after, or in anticipation of loss. Groups can provide companionship, understanding, practical help, a safe place to share feelings, and a place to talk away from overburdened family and friends. Groups can be a safe place for members to draw feelings to the surface so that they can move through to healing, no matter what the outcome of their disease.

Understanding How People Move from Loss to Healing[14]

Any loss that causes a significant change to our lives is a life loss. Death is the most obvious life loss, whether it be the death of parents, children, relatives, friends, or colleagues. But other losses can be wrenching enough to cause pain or grief. These life losses might include the loss of a relationship, a job, a pet, a home, a business, our health, our mobility, or our memory. The loss of a breast or part of a breast from cancer is a life loss. The loss of our sense of power or immortality often accompanies a cancer diagnosis.

The losses and gains people experience when moving through changes from illness or grief can include a loss or gain of any of the following:

---

[14] Caplan S, Lang G. *Grief's Courageous Journey, A Workbook.* Oakland, CA: New Harbinger Publications, 1995.

Living with Breast Cancer

- Self-esteem,
- Control,
- Identity,
- Meaning,
- Belonging, and
- The future.

When grieving or mourning, the feelings that are often present are powerlessness, fear, anger, and guilt. In other words, on the inside we might feel like we are going crazy. This is one of the most common expressions we have heard from bereaved people: "I thought I was going crazy."

Meanwhile, on the outside, certain definite but unwritten rules are taking effect. These rules come from friends, family, workplace, culture, and religion:

The "Unwritten" Rules About Death

- Don't talk about it.

- Don't feel. Don't cry. Don't show emotions. You will upset others.

- Don't trust. This one comes from inside you when you accept the first two rules. "If I cannot feel or talk about it, who can I trust with my feelings, my story, my urge to talk?"

- Don't think for yourself. When you are grieving, you can feel helpless about the loss. This feeling can expand to everything, and you can become vulnerable and open to others telling you what is good and right for you, instead of trusting your own knowledge and instincts.

- Don't change. This is the most dangerous of all. Change is threatening to those around you, because if you can change, then they will have to change. But if you don't change, you won't grow or heal.

So there is pressure from inside: you feel crazy. There is pressure from outside: the rules. What can groups do to help? Groups help break the old rules and develop new ones.

What cancer support groups can do:

- Create a safe place where members tell their story.
- Support members to recognize and manage today's reality.
- Celebrate milestones and members lives.

Anticipatory Grief

Anticipatory grief refers to grieving before the actual loss has occurred. We can anticipate our own death or the death of our group member. We can also anticipate grief associated with the loss of our health, a breast, relationship, job, or sexuality or femininity.

People who are dying can experience anticipatory grief. Usually, however, such grief is experienced by others in the support group and by family members, friends, and caregivers.

Anticipatory grief also allows the grieving person to:

- Absorb the reality of loss over a gradual period of time,
- Finish unfinished business (feelings, unresolved conflicts) with the person,
- Celebrate the life of the person while she is still alive,
- Ask for and give forgiveness,
- Begin to change assumptions about life and identity, and
- Talk to the person who is dying about her plans for how she wants to be remembered, her funeral or memorial service.

The signs of anticipatory grief include:

- Depression,
- Rehearsal of death,
- Heightened concern for the dying person, and
- Attempts to adjust to the consequences of the death.

Transition Cycle

It may be helpful for members of a support group to understand that each of us will experience different emotions at different stages of grief and that these emotions affect us not just once but many times and in no predictable order. Although no one can predict when each of us is ready to move on or where we might be in the cycle, it is helpful to know what behaviors are most commonly expressed at different stages and how group members can be supportive. This diagram illustrates the flow of emotions and different stages that people move through in the process of grief.

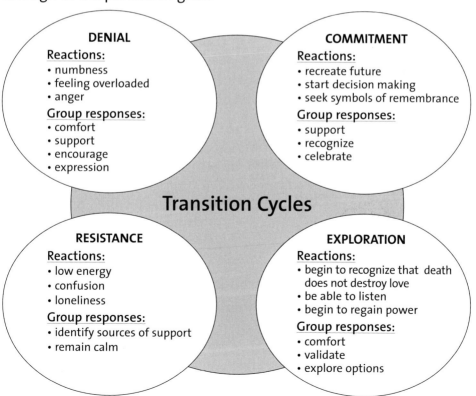

DENIAL

Reactions:
- numbness
- feeling overloaded
- anger

Group responses:
- comfort
- support
- encourage
- expression

COMMITMENT

Reactions:
- recreate future
- start decision making
- seek symbols of remembrance

Group responses:
- support
- recognize
- celebrate

Transition Cycles

RESISTANCE

Reactions:
- low energy
- confusion
- loneliness

Group responses:
- identify sources of support
- remain calm

EXPLORATION

Reactions:
- begin to recognize that death does not destroy love
- be able to listen
- begin to regain power

Group responses:
- comfort
- validate
- explore options

Again, not everyone experiences all of the stages, and people do not move through them in any particular order.

Mourning a Loss

Mourning is a process we go through to help us undo our connection with what we have lost. Mourning helps us to move forward and away from the pain of grief. Mourning rituals such as funerals, burials, and wakes have roots in the cultures and communities we come from. When we experience illness, aging, or a life crisis, we often reach back to our family, culture, or community for help. Rituals help us to recognize, validate, and honor the meaning in each life.

Some groups may decide to acknowledge a member's death by lighting a candle at the beginning of a meeting, standing quietly in a circle, or taking turns reading aloud from a book of affirmations. The practice of using rituals for mourning can help us to gain a sense of being connected to others and reduce our sense of confusion and isolation. Meaningful rituals for mourning offer a sense of comfort, peace, and acceptance in difficult times.

> When a person is born, we celebrate; when they marry we jubilate; but when they die we act as if nothing has happened.
>
> MARGARET MEAD

Final Thoughts: The Trapeze Artist

The trapeze artist can be a symbol of the healing process of grief; we swing back and forth during the grieving period. We hold on to the memories, the legacy of goodness passed on to us—the bonds of love and connection—while letting go of whatever creates bondage and keeps us from moving on, such as guilt, resentment, bitterness, and the inability to forgive either ourselves or others. Keep in mind that we are what connects the past to the future. Like the trapeze artist, we let go of one swing, having faith that we will find and grasp the next swing that will bring us into a whole new experience. Trapezing is an art; it takes practice to find our own natural rhythms and to gain the confidence to let go of one swing and take the bold new action of reaching for the next swing at precisely the right moment.

Living with Breast Cancer

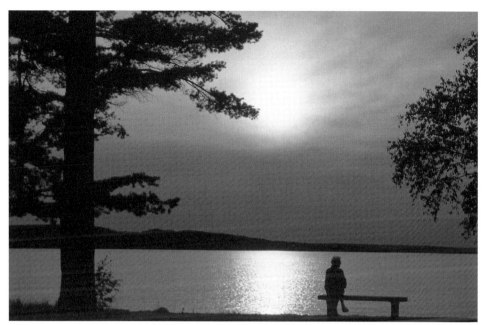

The art of letting go and holding on is a lifetime process of healing. Be gentle with yourself and members of your group because each of you will be at different stages in the grief process. You may at times feel like you and your group members need to move on and get back to normal. It is important to know that you and your group <u>are</u> getting on with life and that the "old normal" is gone forever. You are in a time of transition. It is a gradual building toward a new normal state.

You and other members of your group may at times feel empty. Do not rush in to try and fill up the emptiness. This is the neutral zone, a time of waiting. This time is similar to the changes of seasons—like autumn when the leaves are gone and silence seems to be all around. A waiting time comes; it is a time to rest before new life and new energy appears.

- Grief is a process of change and movement away from the immediate crisis of suffering and loss.

- Grief is a journey without a map or a straight line from beginning to end.

- There are many ways to move from loss to healing and mourning rituals can help.

- Groups can provide help during the grieving journey.

CHAPTER 9

Using Humor

What you can expect to learn in this chapter:
- How laughter can help members connect.
- How humor can provide a balance to the seriousness of a cancer group.
- Appropriate uses of humor.

THE NIGHTLY RITUAL

I prop my wig on the dresser

And tuck my prosthesis beneath

And thank God, I still go to bed with

My man and my very own teeth!

BY JANET HENRY[15]

Many people have described the importance of laughter during group meetings. It is as if laughter provides a balance to the darkness of the cancer experience, as well as a way to connect with others. A good meeting is often described as one with a lot of laughter. The ability of group members to laugh and use humor enhances the work of any support group.

Over 30 years ago, Norman Cousins discovered something we are just beginning to fully realize: laughter can help us heal. In 1964, Cousins, the editor of Saturday Review, was diagnosed with ankylosing spondylitis, a life-threatening illness. His doctors told him he probably wouldn't live. Cousins became very depressed and frustrated while in the hospital and started to take charge of his own treatment—including laughing. The whole time he was sick he used humor so that the positive feelings he got while laughing could strengthen his immune

---

[15] Wooten P. *Compassionate Laughter*, Jest for Your Health. Salt Lake City, UT: Commune-A-Key Publishing, 1996.

system. Not only did he recover, but he found his calling. As Cousins explained in his book, <u>Anatomy of An Illness as Perceived by a Patient</u>, hearty laughter is like vigorous exercise:

> It causes huffing and puffing, speeds up the heart rate, raises blood pressure, increases oxygen consumption, gives the muscles of the face and stomach a workout and relaxes other muscles.[16]

According to researchers Lee Berk and Stanley Tan at California's Loma Linda University "Mirthful laughter induces chemical, molecular benefits throughout our whole body. When you say 'I feel good all over,' that makes a lot of sense. We are capable of influencing our biochemistry by our mood. The evidence keeps piling up; it's just that we've only just started paying attention recently."

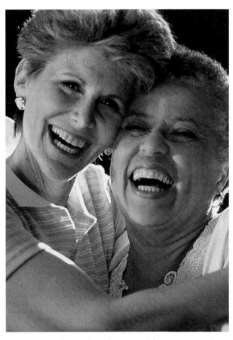

Now that the idea of humor as healing has caught on, there are a number of ways that cancer groups have begun to spread the word to members. Loretta LaRoche, who lectures extensively on the curative powers of humor, has a D.M.A. ("Doesn't mean anything") and teaches that "life is not a dress rehearsal." LaRoche is an adjunct member of the Mind/Body Medical Institute, an affiliate of the Harvard Medical School, and speaks to countless groups about using humor and reducing stress. Her videos are used in many hospitals and she is the author of <u>RELAX—You May Only Have a Few Minutes Left</u>. *"The science is all well and good"* says LaRoche. *"This is a society that thrives on facts. 'If we can up our killer T cells, we just might start laughing.' But you know it's just common sense that laughter works. Laughter is connected to joy, which is connected to gratefulness. 'Gratefulness at being alive.'"*[17]

---

[16] Cousins N. *Anatomy of an illness as perceived by a patient.* New York: W.W. Norton, 1979.

[17] LaRoche L. *RELAX—You may only have a few minutes left: Using the power of humor to overcome stress in your life and work.* New York, NY: Villard Books, 1998.

How to Introduce Humor into Cancer Groups

Used appropriately, humor can be an effective way to build positive relationships between members and improve the spirit in your group. But telling jokes isn't something that everyone is confident doing. Humor is tricky after all; a light touch is essential. There are literally thousands of other ways to encourage laughter and joyful feelings. Here are a few suggestions for using humor:

- One of the simplest ways to use healing laughter is through storytelling. Set the tone by modeling your ability to "tell stories on yourself" whenever appropriate. One participant attended an event and told this story:

  Rose was attending a very serious medical conference. She was feeling out-of-place because it seemed that everyone in attendance was a doctor— using a beeper or a cell phone or a lap top computer. Rose was "beeper less" and feeling very unimportant. So, she went home that night, and came back the next day to the conference with a big smile on her face...wearing her garage door opener.

  JOEL GOODMAN, THE HUMOR PROJECT, SARATOGA SPRINGS, NEW YORK

- Build humor into your group culture or spirit. For example, some hospitals now have humor carts or humor rooms with toys, games, jokes, and videos for patients and staff. Include some humorous books or joke books in your group library.

- Remember to use humor as a tool, not a weapon. Laughing with others builds confidence, brings people together, and pokes fun at our common dilemmas. Laughing at others destroys confidence, erodes teamwork, and embarrasses others. Use humor to help build connections in groups.

Loretta LaRoche[17] also suggests the following ideas for using humor:

- *Buy something silly and wear it. A Groucho Marx mustache and glasses are my favorite. Put them on in situations where you tend to see only the worst outcome. I wear mine when I drive through Boston, especially when I have to merge. People always let me in.*

- *Write down your favorite profanities and then assign each of them a number. If someone is getting on your nerves, don't curse; just say the number. They'll never know. When they walk by, say "four."*

- *Be in the moment. Don't put off your happiness or your life for a better time. There's a saying that I often use to close my lectures: Yesterday is history. Tomorrow is a mystery. And today is a gift. That's why they call it the present.*

A Word of Caution

Humor has its place, but there are times when it is not appropriate to use. A time when humor should not be used is during a serious conversation. Another time might be when someone is using humor to avoid discussing difficult emotions or to try and hide hostility or anger. Humor used in this way does not help. When this happens, the group needs to bring the focus back to the difficult issue being discussed.

Final Thoughts

Something to help *you* experience the benefits of humor.

Things I Learned From My Dog[18]

- Never pass up the opportunity for a joyride.
- When a loved one comes home, always run to greet them.
- When it's in your best interest, practice obedience.
- Take naps and stretch before rising.
- Run, romp, and play daily.
- Eat with gusto and enthusiasm.
- Be loyal.
- Never pretend to be something you're not.
- If what you want lies buried, dig until you find it.
- When someone is having a bad day, be silent, sit close, and nuzzle them.
- Thrive on attention and let people touch you.
- Avoid biting when a simple growl will do.
- On hot days, drink plenty of water and lay under a shady tree.
- When you're happy, dance around and wag your body.
- Bond with your pack.
- Delight in the joy of a long walk.

KEY MESSAGE FROM THIS CHAPTER:

- Practice telling stories on yourself, use humor, laugh, and stay well.

---

[18]Wooten P. *Compassionate Laughter*, Jest for Your Health.

CHAPTER 10

Planning and Evaluation with Your Group

What you can expect to learn about in this chapter:
- How to recognize and use the natural cycles of a group for planning.
- Characteristics of successful groups.
- How to evaluate the effectiveness of a self-help group.

Group Seasons and Cycles

There is a cyclical, seasonal, and predictable nature to the life cycle of groups. Although a diagnosis of breast cancer can happen at anytime, interest in joining or participating in a group seems to have a pattern or cycle. The cycle often parallels the school year. Beginning in the fall, group members will feel a surge in energy and renewed attendance. Your group can use this to help develop a year-long planning cycle. In this way, your group members won't feel as if they need to do everything at once, and you may not be so overwhelmed when demands start adding up!

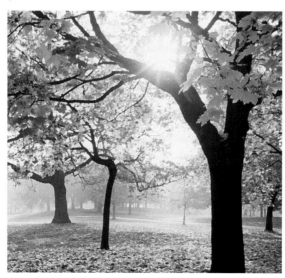

Planning

Fall is often a good time to talk about planning any special events or speakers and for members to change or stop doing some jobs or take on new ones. You might also want to think about planning special activities during April (Cancer Awareness Month), June (National Cancer Survivor's Day), and October (Breast Cancer Awareness Month). Your group may want to plan to schedule a time for reviewing the role of the facilitators and invite other group members to consider learning the skills necessary to assume this role. Plan to participate in training and skill-building workshops such as those for group facilitators. Experienced facilitators can also plan ways to coach and mentor new people until they gain the skills and confidence they need.

If your group has a budget, find out what conferences or events your members want to attend during the year and plan for these expenses. If you decide to start projects such as a newsletter or fundraising events, you will need to find volunteers and start planning early. Some groups will plan a date for ceremonies to remember and celebrate the lives of members.

September, January, and June are also the times many groups reflect on or evaluate group meetings. Think about what is working well and ask members if their needs and expectations are being met.

Evaluation

On a quarterly basis, it will be helpful to take stock of what is working for your members and what isn't. It is normal in any group for things to sometimes come to a standstill. Members may become bored, frustrated, lacking in energy, less committed, or less interested in other issues. If members expect one thing from the group and are getting something else, they may leave or become frustrated. When members are leaving and you don't know why, an evaluation can help your group understand why members leave and what, if anything, the group needs to do. Evaluation is a process for measuring what is working for your group and what needs changing. It is not a judgment about success or failure.

Evaluation is also a way to recognize and reward facilitators for their time and effort. When a group provides special recognition for the work of the facilitators, the group will help prevent burnout.

You might be wondering what a group should be doing in order to be effective for members. Effective cancer self-help groups are described as[19]:

- Accepting,
- Cooperative,
- Warm,
- Friendly and welcoming,
- Confidential,
- Demonstrating shared decision making,
- Demonstrating open communication,
- Diverse,
- Nonjudgmental,
- Having few rules,
- Everyone knowing the purpose of the group,
- Energetic,
- Using humor, and
- Trusting.

You might ask members to discuss the list of characteristics and consider how your group is doing in these areas. This can help identify places that need work or where members may have skills that can be used to improve your meetings.

Some groups wait until the group is really in trouble before they sit down and try to understand what is happening. Ongoing evaluation that is planned and a part of the normal activities for your group is one way to ensure that the group has clear goals and that the goals are being achieved. Evaluation should not interfere with the group or be threatening in any way.

---

[19] Cella DF, Sarafian B, Snider PR, Yellen SB, Winicour P. Evaluation of a community-based cancer support group. *Journal of Psycho-Oncology* 1993;2:123 – 132.

How to Measure Success

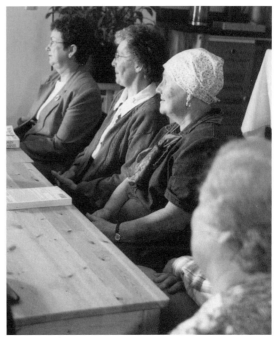

There are several ways to do an evaluation. The group can have a candid discussion about group goals and agreements, or members can be asked to fill out a short evaluation form. An experienced outside observer can sit in on a group meeting and describe the process as she sees it. Your group should plan to do an evaluation about two to three times each year. The purpose of each evaluation is to find out if members have received the support, information, and guidance they expected. You can also ask members how joining the group has affected their relationships with friends, family, and doctors.

Group Discussion and Confidential Evaluation Forms

Groups can begin with an open discussion about the purpose of the evaluation, what the process will be, and how the information will be used and then ask members to complete a confidential evaluation form (Appendix C). The process will require a group member to act as a leader or facilitator for the discussion. If the group members will also be commenting on the facilitation process, ask someone other than the regular facilitators to lead the discussion or have the members complete a confidential evaluation form. Otherwise, some members will be uncomfortable talking about the work of the facilitators. The group discussion can be recorded on a flip chart and the individual evaluations can be summarized and ideas brought back to the group at a later time. If members have made suggestions for changing the meetings or ground rules, these ideas will need to be discussed before changes are made. The individual evaluation forms and the record of the discussions can be used to plan changes.

The following are some suggestions for discussion questions:

- What were you expecting to get when you first joined the group?
- What is one thing you appreciate about the group?
- How do you view your own participation?
- How do you feel about the role you have played?
- Describe a good experience you remember in the group.
- Describe one thing you would like to have happen in the group.
- Describe a gift or skill you bring to the group.
- Describe what you understand the purpose of the group to be.

Once your members have completed the evaluation process, use the findings about what is working and what needs to change. Brainstorm ideas about how to make those changes happen. Set out a plan and timetable and indicate who is responsible for the actions or activities. Report back to your group about the evaluation and the planning activities. Keep a record of the evaluation and plans in the group journal. When members know what changes are coming up, they will feel involved and their sense of belonging with the group will increase. Planning and informing members about planned changes can help you to avoid anxiety over sudden changes to the meeting location or schedule or having new facilitators.

Consider measuring your success by such things as:

- Members giving and getting support through regular group meetings.
- Veteran members helping women who are newly diagnosed.
- Members "graduating" from the group and feeling they got what they needed.

- Groups often operate to the rhythm of seasonal cycles.

- Planning is needed to keep the group organized and active.

- A periodic review of the meetings allows members to reflect on the strengths and weaknesses of the group's work.

- Evaluation helps the group to understand how the group is succeeding and whether changes are needed.

CHAPTER 11

As Your Group Grows and Changes

What you can expect to learn about in this chapter:
- How to find and build on the strengths of other groups with a shared interest.
- How to network with other self-help groups.
- How to develop relationships with health care professionals and institutions.
- How to use the media to promote your group.

As your group grows and changes, it will attract women from other groups, health care professionals and providers, and the media. This chapter provides some ideas on how to deal with these groups.

Finding and Building on the Strengths of Other Self-Help Groups

Your group may want to network with other cancer self-help groups for a lot of reasons:

- To share resources,
- To get advice or coaching when the group is getting started,
- To build coalitions for fund raising or advocacy,
- To attend workshops together,
- To learn different perspectives,
- To support one another through difficult times,
- To build confidence,
- To educate the public, and
- To collaborate on projects.

Even if your cancer self-help group does not want formal partnerships with other cancer groups or organizations, you will likely meet people from other groups, especially if you are doing community outreach or working on committees or boards that provide cancer care services.

Networking with Other Self-Help Groups

If your group is interested in learning about other self-help groups, here are some tips on how you could network with them and stay in touch:

- Get in touch with other group facilitators and ask how you might share ideas, provide support or encouragement for each other, or work together on projects.
- Attend each other's meetings as guests.
- Find opportunities for joint meetings, retreats, and workshop training.
- Get together by telephone or letter to give each other moral support and share skills.
- Have a joint group meeting on a common issue and invite a guest speaker.
- Start a joint newsletter.

Networking with Agencies and Cancer Care Institutions

- Invite nurses, oncologists, or other cancer experts to come as guest speakers.
- Offer to speak at the institution about your group.
- Seek opportunities for joint workshops or advocacy efforts.
- Plan joint activities or ask them to sponsor guest speakers that interest both groups.
- Offer to write an article or put an insert about your group in their newsletter.

Living with Breast Cancer

Developing Good Relationships with Health Care Providers

Groups may want to develop good relationships with health care providers because they value professional participation or because it may increase access to resources and expertise. Professional support can give your group more credibility, especially with policy makers and others. Professionals also value self-help groups as a way of helping their patients get emotional support and practical help in dealing with their concerns.

Your group may want to consider the following ideas for building relationships with professionals:

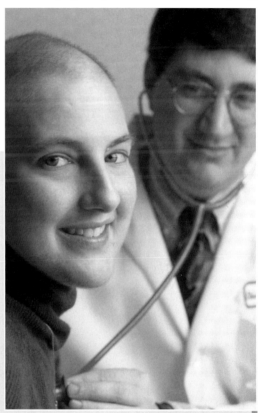

© Leif Skoogfors/CORBIS/MAGMA

- Invite nurses, oncologists, or other cancer experts to come to your group as guest speakers.

- Offer to talk at hospitals, clinics, or cancer centers about your group.

- Plan joint activities or ask the hospital or cancer center to sponsor guest speakers of interest to both groups.

- Offer to write an article or put an insert about your group in their newsletter.

Whatever the nature of the relationship between self-help groups and cancer care professionals, there must be mutual respect, tolerance, and understanding of each other's roles and commitment in order for the relationship to work.

TIPS:

✓ *Choose professionals who share common values with your group.*

✓ *Learn about potential partners before making a decision to work together.*

✓ *Decide what the purpose and goals of the partnership will be.*

✓ *Follow up contacts with a call or letter.*

✓ *Keep a file of the contacts and information shared.*

✓ *Educate professionals about the benefits of cancer self-help groups.*

✓ *Evaluate your relationships and outcomes from time to time.*

Promoting Your Group and Developing Effective Relationships with the Media

Working with the media may or may not be something your group wants to do. However, cancer is a very popular topic in the media and human interest stories about people living with the disease are often used to explain the importance of new discoveries and treatments. You should be prepared to answer questions in the way your group wants to be represented. When you promote your group, you should be able to describe your group well, including the group history, goals, meetings, and contact person. In order to reach potential members, you will also need to promote and advertise your group in hospitals, doctors' offices, and counselors' offices and to social workers.

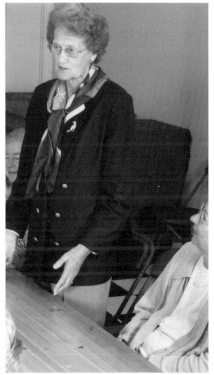

TIPS:

✓ *Identify and know your message. Get group consensus on how you want to describe your group and be consistent with the messages.*

✓ *Get to know the media. Try to get to know individuals from TV, radio, newspapers, magazines, and other media. Set up a meeting and introduce your group.*

✓ *Have a knowledgeable, designated spokesperson.*

✓ *Use the media to reach your real audience.*

✓ *Be prepared. Use only facts that you know are current and from reliable sources such as the National Cancer Institute. When the media interviews you about your group or issue, they assume that you know what you are talking about. Do some research and be prepared. Don't pretend to know something you don't. Admit it and ask if you can get back to them with an answer. Then do it.*

✓ *Make clear guidelines about confidentiality for your group.*

✓ *Stay focused and get your message across clearly.*

Closing

As breast cancer survivors, we are seeking new ways to heal and to learn to live with disease—to look everywhere for effective ways to bring meaning and vitality into our lives. After many years of being involved with self-help groups, we still love what we do, and we still gain tremendous satisfaction from enriching the lives of other women living with breast cancer.

In this guide, we hope that we have given you some explanations about what breast cancer self-help groups can do and what the research has to say, as well as some ideas on how to start and maintain effective groups. As we said in the beginning, our intention in writing this was to provide some direction and encouragement for your work.

All of us who are involved with breast cancer have a role to play in ensuring that women know about the support that is available through self-help groups. All women affected need to know about the unique and powerful source of support and information that is available in their community.

Family doctors, cancer clinics, and hospitals can help you to reach women who are searching for the support of others. They can also help to ensure that your group is listed in the resource directories for cancer patients and health professionals.

Spread the word about the wonderful work your group is doing and celebrate your achievements in your community! Celebrate together— your lives and your work!

Understanding Your Own Group Behavior: A Personal Skills Inventory[20]

Another way you can help yourself to understand if you are well suited to the job of starting or facilitating a self-help group is to think about the ways in which you have behaved in other groups. Read through the choices in the following lists and decide where you fit on the scale. Then review your list and choose the skills you want to work on.

COMMUNICATION	OK	NEED TO DO MORE	NEED TO DO LESS
Talking in groups			
Being brief and concise			
Drawing out others			
Listening generously			
Thinking before speaking			
Keeping my comments on the topic			
Not interrupting			

OBSERVATION SKILLS	OK	NEED TO DO MORE	NEED TO DO LESS
Being aware of tension in the group			
Being aware of the energy level			
Being aware of who is talking to whom			
Being aware of the interest level			
Sensing the feelings			
Being aware of who is not talking			
Being aware of anyone who is left out			
Being aware of the effect my comments have on others			
Being aware of the group avoiding or distracting			
Being aware of silences			

[20] Town C. *Towards Effective Self-Help—A Group Facilitation Training Manual*. Hamilton, ON: Prevention Network of Hamilton-Wentworth, 1993. Adapted with permission.

PROBLEM SOLVING SKILLS	OK	NEED TO DO MORE	NEED TO DO LESS
Recognizing a problem			
Stating problems clearly			
Asking for ideas, opinions, responses			
Giving ideas			
Summarizing the discussion			
Clarifying the issues			
Making a decision			
Implementing the decision			

MORALE BUILDING SKILLS	OK	NEED TO DO MORE	NEED TO DO LESS
Showing interest			
Getting others involved			
Creating linkages			
Getting agreement			
Ensuring safe, democratic, open process			
Appreciating/recognizing individual contributions			

EMOTIONAL EXPRESSIVENESS	OK	NEED TO DO MORE	NEED TO DO LESS
Telling others how I genuinely feel			
Hiding my emotions			
Disagreeing openly			
Expressing warmth			
Expressing gratitude			
Being sarcastic			

FACING AND ACCEPTING EMOTIONAL SITUATIONS	OK	NEED TO DO MORE	NEED TO DO LESS
Facing conflict and anger			
Facing closeness and affection			
Accepting silence			
Facing disappointment/sadness			
Facing grief or loss			

SOCIAL RELATIONSHIPS	OK	NEED TO DO MORE	NEED TO DO LESS
Acting dominant			
Trusting others			
Being helpful			
Being protective			
Rescuing			
Needing attention on me			
Standing up for myself			

GENERAL	OK	NEED TO DO MORE	NEED TO DO LESS
Understanding why I do what I do (insight)			
Encouraging feedback from others about my behavior			
Accepting help willingly			
Giving feedback to others			
Criticizing myself			
Waiting patiently			

Appendix B

Self-Help Research

The following information can be helpful to health care professionals and facilitators or group leaders who are interested in research about the effectiveness of self-help groups. It may also be helpful if you are explaining self-help to someone outside your group.

> Self-help groups are a powerful and constructive means for people to help themselves and each other. The basic dignity of each human being is expressed in his or her capacity to be involved in a reciprocal helping exchange. Out of this compassion comes cooperation. From this cooperation comes community. With the increased awareness and understanding of these groups, the number of mutual help communities will continue to grow—and continue to provide their members with the direction, values and hope they need. In a sense, they speak for all of us since even those of us who study these groups as research professionals are consumers.[21]

For the past few decades, researchers have been evaluating the effects of self-help/mutual aid groups for participants. Most research studies of self-help groups have found some benefits of participation. The purpose of providing the information that follows is to briefly summarize some of the research supporting the effectiveness of self-help groups.

Unfortunately, the research on the effects of self-help groups is confusing. Many studies that claim to evaluate self-help groups are actually studies of psychotherapy or support groups solely led by professionals who do not share the condition shared by the group. We have tried to focus on groups where the participants all had cancer and ran the group on their own. We included studies where a group was co-led by a professional and a self-helper or where the model of group facilitation had lessons for self-helpers. Professional involvement did not rule a study out of consideration because, in the real world, many member-run self-help groups use professional advisors.

---

[21] Silverman P. *The Self-Help Source Book: Finding and Forming Mutual Aid Self-Help Groups.* American Self-Help Clearinghouse, 1996.

Maisiak R, Cain M. Evaluation of TOUCH: an oncology self-help group. <u>Oncology Nursing Forum</u> 1981;8(3):20 – 25

This study surveyed 139 members of TOUCH, a self-help group for cancer patients in Alabama. TOUCH focuses on teaching its members about cancer and training them to be peer counselors to help other patients. The longer members participated in a group, the more they improved their knowledge of cancer, their ability to talk with others, friendships, family life, coping with the disease, and following of doctor's orders. The percentage of people indicating that their coping was very good after TOUCH was 59%, more than double the percentage indicating that it was very good before TOUCH (28%).

Spiegel D, Bloom JR, Kraemer HC, Gottheil E. Effect of psychosocial treatment on survival of patients with metastatic breast cancer. <u>The Lancet</u> October 1989;14:888 – 891.

Participants in this study were 86 women undergoing treatment for metastatic breast cancer. A subset of these women (50) was randomly assigned to have their oncologic care supplemented with a weekly support group. The support groups were co-facilitated by a therapist who had breast cancer in remission and a psychiatrist or social worker. The sessions focused on living life fully, improving communication with family members and doctors, facing death, expressing emotions such as grief, and controlling pain through self-hypnosis. On average, support group participants lived twice as long as those who did not participate in groups.

Heiney SP, Wells LM. Strategies for organizing and maintaining successful support groups. <u>Oncology Nursing Forum</u> 1989;16:803 – 809.

Nurses often become involved in organizing and leading support groups either through their own institutions or at the request of consumers interested in starting self-help groups. Nurses without formal training in group therapy may find it difficult to organize and maintain support groups. Successful strategies, based on group therapy techniques and project management skills, can assist group leaders in organizing a group "from scratch" or in revitalizing existing groups.

This article describes the strategies that help in organizing and maintaining groups for people with cancer and their families.

Cella DF, Sarafian B, Snider PR, et al. Evaluation of a community-based cancer support group. Journal of Psycho-Oncology, 1993;2:123 – 132.

This paper provides process and outcome data from 77 people with cancer who completed an 8-week support group facilitated by licenced and trained mental health professionals in a local community cancer support organization. Similar to the experience of others, participants were primarily female, of European descent, well educated, and relatively young (mean age of 50). As predicted, their self-reported quality of life improved significantly. Ratings of the group and the facilitator were consistently and strikingly positive. Although facilitators were rated positively and appreciated for their presence, peer support exceeded facilitator skill/input as the primary ingredient noted by participants to be the most helpful aspect of the group. Community-based support groups appear to provide measurable benefit to participants who complete the group. The benefit is consistent with that demonstrated in randomized studies and emphasizes improvement in coping stimulated by mutual support in a safe environment.

Cella DF, Yellen SB. Cancer support groups: the state of the art. Cancer Practice 1993;1:1 – 6.

Support groups serve a large number of people with cancer and their family members. Their popularity is grounded in the fact that the existing cancer treatment network continues to leave a gap of unmet psychosocial needs. These unmet needs can often be alleviated by mutual aid provided by people who share a common experience. Mutual aid complements professional help by adding a dimension of support that is best provided by other members of the group in need. Themes of discussion in support groups include the emotional impact of illness, family difficulty, problems of intimacy, sense of isolation/stigma, role changes, and cancer-specific concerns. Components of mutual aid include direct assistance, advice giving, and emotional support. In cancer support groups, there is an under-representation of people of color, men, and the poor among group participants. Outreach to underserved groups must include more creative and flexible helping mechanisms.

Phillips C, Gray RE, Davis C, Fitch M. What breast cancer self-help groups want you to know. <u>Canadian Family Physician</u> 1996;42: 1447 – 1449.

Researchers interested in women's involvement in breast cancer self-help groups studied groups in four communities. The groups ranged in size from 10 to 35 regular participants of all ages and all stages of breast cancer. The groups were led by breast cancer survivors and not professionals. In each group, members expressed frustration about the medical community's lack of interest in understanding the ways in which women are helped by these groups. Many women believe that their physicians look skeptically at their involvement, and a few report that their physicians see the groups as potentially harmful. What explains this scepticism about the value of self-help groups? Some physicians underestimate the psychosocial needs of their patients, whereas others are wary of recommending groups about which they know little.

The paper outlines some concerns physicians have raised with members and the members response to them.

Gray R, Fitch M, Davis C, Phillips C. A qualitative study of breast cancer self-help groups. <u>Journal of Psycho-Oncology</u> 1997;6:279 – 289.

This study reports on the experience of women in four community breast cancer self-help groups in Ontario, Canada. Interviews were conducted with 24 women about the benefits and limitations of their group involvement and about their perspectives on group processes and structures. Overall, participants reported their group involvement to be extremely helpful for navigating the short- and long-term impact of breast cancer. Emotional support benefits included connecting with other breast cancer survivors, feeling understood and sharing experiences, providing hope, and sharing healing laughter. Informational and practical support benefits included sharing important information and learning how to get what you want. Even where there were concerns about limitations or tensions of group experience, these occurred against a backdrop of appreciation and committment. From the discussion of group processes and structures, a number of issues were identified as problematic. Most notable were how to deal with deaths of members and how to balance the group's primary purpose of providing support with secondary goals of dealing with group business and engaging in meaningful advocacy.

Gray RE, Carroll JC, Fitch M, et al. Cancer self-help groups and family physicians. Cancer Practice 1991;7(1):10 – 15.

Despite the phenomenal growth during the past decade of cancer self-help groups, little research has been conducted to document the relationship between groups and health care professionals, especially physicians. This study provides information about family physician practices and awareness and attitudes about self-help groups.

RESEARCH ON SOCIAL SUPPORT AND MORTALITY

There is general agreement in health and social sciences research that social support for people with serious illness "works." A landmark 9-year study of 7,000 people in Alameda, California, considered four types of social ties—marriage, relationships with parents and close friends, membership in a religious group, and membership in other groups—to identify a link between social support and health. In every health category, people with many social networks had lower mortality rates over the 9 years (Hammer, 1985).

RESEARCH ON SOCIAL SUPPORT AND WOMEN WITH BREAST CANCER[22]

Several studies have identified a relationship between social support and a woman's quality of life while she is living with breast cancer. Strong social and family networks are associated with fewer emotional disruptions (Johnson and Lane, 1993), lower levels of anxiety and depression (Neuling, 1988; Primomo and Yates, 1990), and decreased isolation and alienation (Spiegel et al., 1989). Other studies suggest

---

[22] Hands on Help: A Manual for Breast Cancer Self Help and Mutual Support Groups.
The Breast Cancer Support Network for Ontario Project, Burlington, ON, 1996.

that social support may be linked to the delayed spread or recurrence of disease (Levy, 1990) and to longer survival (Johnson, 1993; Maunsell, 1995; Spiegel et al., 1989; Waxler-Morrison and Hislop, 1991).

A study in British Columbia of the effect of social relationships on survival for 133 women with breast cancer found that women's friendships, social networks, and employment were significantly related to survival; the extent to which a woman felt that she could call upon three or more friends for support or help was most strongly associated with survival (Waxler-Morrison and Hislue, 1991).

There is surprisingly little systemic research on self-help groups despite years of clinical and policy interest (Gray, 1991). Yet improvements in quality of life as a result of participation in a support group has been well demonstrated (Cella and Yellen, 1993).

Gray (1991) cites two studies of cancer self-help groups, one of which indicated that group participation had resulted in increased knowledge of cancer, increased sense of life's meaningfulness, and increased ability to cope with illness. In another study, people interviewed indicated that the group had allowed them to gain a better perspective on illness, heightened self-awareness, an increased ability to talk about cancer, and improved self-image (Gray, 1991). Spiegel's study of self-help groups demonstrated the value to cancer patients of these groups in reducing isolation.

The opportunity to measure one's own experience against another's and the opportunity to observe how others have coped (to adopt role models) and help with clarifying problems are benefits of meeting and speaking with people who have the same disease (Cella and Yellen, 1993).

Waxler-Morrison and Hislop (1991) point to the importance of women with breast cancer having a support network beyond their immediate families. Family relationships may be ambivalent or conflictual, and many women hide the extent of their fears or pain from their relatives; members of a more distant network, although providing less support, may be able to provide support that is more satisfactory and more meaningful. Benefits, then, that accrue from the opportunity for a complete "telling of the story" and the chance to be honest and direct about pain and fear occur in the context of mutual support groups. Improved communication with family and friends is thought to result from support group participation.

An increase in social and physical activity is also cited as a benefit of mutual support group participation, as is increased ability to cope with medical procedures.

Reissman identifies the "helper therapy principle" to account for some of the benefits that participants in mutual support groups derive from their provision of support to other members. These include increased level of interpersonal competence as a result of making an impact on another's life, valuable personalized learning, and social approval (Killilea, 1976).

RESEARCH ON SELF-HELP GROUP PARTICIPANTS: RELATIONSHIPS TO MEDICAL SYSTEM

People who get support have a higher level of well-being, so they may be less susceptible to fatigue, stress and illness. Mutual support or self-help groups provide opportunities for information sharing about illness and skills for coping. As well, women who experience improvements in their communication skills may be better able to access information and treatment from professionals.

References

Cella D, Yellen S. Cancer support groups: the state of the art. Cancer Practice 1993;1(1):56 – 61.

Hammer M. Core and extended social networks in relation to health and wellness. Social Science and Medicine 1985;17:405 – 411.

Johnson J, Lane C. Role of support groups in cancer care. Supportive Care Cancer 1993;1:52 – 56.

Killilea M. Support Systems and Mutual Help. New York: Grune and Stratton, 1976.

Maunsell E. Social support and survival among women with breast cancer. Cancer 1995;76:631 – 637.

McLean B. Social support, support groups and breast cancer: a literature review. Canadian Journal of Community Mental Health 1995;14:207 – 227.

Neuling S. Social support and recovery after surgery for breast cancer: frequency and correlates of supportive behaviours by family, friends, and surgeons. Social Science and Medicine 1988;27:385 – 382.

Primomo J, Yates B. Social support for women during chronic illness: the relationship among sources and types to adjustment. Research in nursing and health. Ottawa: Canadian Council on Social Development, 1990.

Spiegel D, Bloom J, Kraemer J. Effects of Psychosocial treatment on survival of patients with metastatic breast cancer. The Lancet 1989;2:888 – 891.

Waxler-Morrison N, Hislop T. Effects of social relationships on survival of women with breast cancer: a prospective study. Social Science and Medicine 1991;33:177 – 183.

Other Research References

Borkman T. Self-help groups at the turning point: emerging egalitarian alliances with the formal health care system? American Journal of Community Psychology 1990;18:321 – 332.

Bradburn J, Maher EJ, Young J, Young T. Community based cancer support groups: an undervalued resource? Clinical Oncology 1992;4: 377 – 380.

Fridinger F, Goodwin G, Chng CI. Physician and consumer attitudes and behaviours regarding self-help health support groups as an adjunct to traditional medical care. Journal of Health and Social Policy 1992;3:19 – 36.

Hitch PJ, Fielding RG, Llewelyn SP. Effectiveness of self-help and support groups for cancer patients: a review. Psychology and Health 1994;9:437 – 448.

Leis AM, Haines CS, Pancyr GC. Exploring oncologists' beliefs about psychosocial groups; implications for patient care and research. Journal of Psychosocial Oncology 1994;12:77 – 87.

Stewart MJ. Professional interface with mutual-aid self-help groups: a review. Social Science Medicine 1990;31:1143 – 1158.

Sample Evaluation Forms

EVALUATION OF SATISFACTION [21]

Date:_____

1. How did you learn about the group?

   ❏ A friend   ❏ Referred by a professional

   ❏ Newspaper   ❏ Other

2. Is this your first meeting?   ❏ Yes   ❏ No

3. Will you attend future meetings? ❏ Yes   ❏ No

4. Please assess the following aspects of the meeting:

	VERY SATISFIED	SOMEWHAT SATISFIED	NOT SATISFIED
Facilitators' skills	❏	❏	❏
Structure of the meeting	❏	❏	❏
Format of the meeting	❏	❏	❏
Length of the meeting	❏	❏	❏
Opportunity to talk	❏	❏	❏
Time of the meeting	❏	❏	❏
Location	❏	❏	❏

5. How helpful was the group for you?

   Not helpful   ❏   Somewhat helpful   ❏

   Very helpful ❏   Extremely helpful ❏

6. Describe briefly what was most helpful to you:

   _____

7. What did you like most about the group meeting?

   _____

---

[21] Adapted with permission from ACS. Guidelines on support and self-help groups. Atlanta, GA: American Cancer Society, 1994.

8. What did you like least about the group?

    _____

9. Do you feel any different about yourself after the group?

    ❏ Yes   ❏ No

    If yes, in what ways do you feel different?

    _____

10. Have you changed any behaviors, ways, or habits since participating in the group?

    ❏ Yes   ❏ No

    If yes, what has changed?

    _____

11. Please comment or provide suggestions for future groups and/or suggestions for improvement.

    _____

    _____

    _____

    _____

    _____

    _____

    _____

    _____

    _____

    _____

THANK YOU.

BREAST CANCER SUPPORT GROUP SATISFACTION SURVEY[22]

Support Group Mission:

> To provide a safe environment for women with breast cancer to share feelings and experiences and obtain support throughout all stages of their treatment: from diagnosis to survival. The goals of the Step at a Time Support Group are to educate, support and link women facing breast cancer with community resources.

Instructions: In an effort to improve the quality of services provided to our patients, it is important to first evaluate the impact of these services on the quality of life of the patients we treat. We are interested in understanding what factors related to the Breast Cancer Support Group have the greatest impact on your ability to cope with a cancer diagnosis. Please complete the following survey and return it in the self-addressed envelope. Your insight will help us to develop educational programs and activities to improve the quality of our services and ensure that the support group meets your individual needs. Thank you for your cooperation.

Age: _____   Date Diagnosed: _____

Type of Cancer: _____

Type of Surgery: _____

Type of Treatment: ❏ Radiation   ❏ Chemotherapy

                             ❏ Surgery   ❏ No Treatment

                             ❏ Other _____

Since your diagnosis, how many times have you attended the breast cancer support group?

            ❏ 0 – 4 times   ❏ 5 – 10 times

            ❏ 10 – 15 times   ❏ more than 15 times

[22] Walsh C. Mission Hospital Regional Medical Center. Used with permission.

1. To what extent does the Breast Cancer Support Group address the physical symptoms associated with your diagnosis and treatment?

   Poor 1   2   3   4   5 Excellent

2. To what degree does the support group address the emotional aspects associated with your diagnosis and treatment?

   Poor 1   2   3   4   5 Excellent

3. How well does the support group address the spiritual aspects associated with your diagnosis and treatment?

   Poor 1   2   3   4   5 Excellent

4. How well does the support group address the impact a cancer diagnosis has on your social interactions?

   Poor 1   2   3   4   5 Excellent

5. How would you rate the staff's ability to facilitate the group and answer questions?

   Poor 1   2   3   4   5 Excellent

6. Please indicate which treatment side effects you experienced while on therapy.

   ❏ Nausea/vomiting   ❏ Concerns about body image

   ❏ Weight change   ❏ Anxiety

   ❏ Hair loss   ❏ Depression

   ❏ Fatigue/weakness   ❏ Change in sleep patterns

   ❏ Appetite problems   ❏ Infection

   ❏ Pain   ❏ Other_____

7. To what degree has the support group helped you manage with treatment side effects?

   Poor 1   2   3   4   5 Excellent

8. On a scale of 1 – 5 (1 = poor and 5 = excellent) rate the effectiveness of the breast cancer support group in addressing quality of life issues.

QUALITY OF LIFE FACTORS	EFFECTIVENESS OF THIS GROUP TO HELP YOU WITH THIS ISSUE				
PAIN	Poor 1	2	3	4	5 Excellent
Ability to do daily activities	Poor 1	2	3	4	5 Excellent
Ability to work in or out of home/go to school	Poor 1	2	3	4	5 Excellent
Interaction with family	Poor 1	2	3	4	5 Excellent
Participate in social activities	Poor 1	2	3	4	5 Excellent
Sexual function/intimacy	Poor 1	2	3	4	5 Excellent
Fear of the future	Poor 1	2	3	4	5 Excellent
Fear of cancer recurrence/relapse	Poor 1	2	3	4	5 Excellent
Emotional well-being	Poor 1	2	3	4	5 Excellent
Financial security/insurance issues	Poor 1	2	3	4	5 Excellent

9. Do you have any suggestions on ways the breast cancer support group can improve its services?

10. We welcome any other comments you would like to make.

THANK YOU FOR YOUR ASSISTANCE.

Resources

- **American Cancer Society**
  1599 Clifton Road, NE
  Atlanta, GA 30329
  800-ACS-2345
  www.cancer.org

The ACS is a national organization with local offices throughout the U.S. It provides information and referrals to numerous local and community support services and maintains a library of cancer education publications available to the public.

- **AMC Cancer Research Center**
  1600 Pier Street
  Denver, CO 80214
  800-525-3777
  www.amc.org

Provides information on symptoms, diagnosis, treatment, psychosocial issues, support groups, and other valuable resources, such as financial aid and transportation services.

- **American Self-Help Clearinghouse**
  St. Clare's Hospital
  25 Pocono Road
  Denville, NJ 07834
  800-367-6274
  Mentalhelp.net/selfhelp

Serves as a guide for exploring support groups and networks within one's community and throughout the world.

- **CancerCare**
  275 7th Avenue
  New York, NY 10001
  800-813-HOPE
  www.cancercare.org

A nonprofit organization providing emotional support, information, and practical help to people with cancer and their families and friends. Helping Hands: The Resource Guide for People with Cancer is available at no extra charge.

- **Cancer Information Service**
  National Cancer Institute (NCI)
  Office of Cancer Communications
  31 Center Dr. MSC 2580
  Bldg. 31, Room 10A03
  Bethesda, MD 20892-2580
  800-4-CANCER
  www.nci.nih.gov

The Cancer Information Service provides up-to-date information on cancer to patients and their families, health professionals, and the general public. Materials can be accessed on the Website or by calling CIS.

- **Intercultural Cancer Council**
  PMB-C
  1720 Dryden
  Houston, TX 77030
  713-798-4617
  www.iccnetwork.org

The Intercultural Cancer Council has developed policies and programs that address the high incidence rates of cancer among minority populations.

- **Mautner Project for Lesbians with Cancer**
  1707 L. St. NW, Suite 500
  Washington, DC 20036
  202-332-5536
  www.mautnerproject.org

This initiative offers education, information, support, advocacy, and direct services for lesbians with cancer and their loved ones.

- **NABCO: National Alliance of Breast Cancer Organizations**
  9 E 37th Street, 10th Fl.
  New York, NY 10016
  212-889-0606
  888-80-NABCO
  www.nabco.org

NABCO is a nonprofit resource that provides up-to-date, accurate information for patients and their families, media, professionals, and medical organizations. It provides a large variety of professionally prepared information resources.

- **National Asian Women's Health organization (NAWHO)**
  250 Montgomery St. Ste. 1500
  San Francisco, CA 94104
  415-989-9747
  www.nawho.org

NAWHO is a nonprofit, community-based health advocacy organization committed to improving the overall health status of Asian women and girls.

- **National Breast Cancer Coalition**
  1707 L Street, NW, Ste. 1060
  Washington, DC 20036
  202-296-7477
  www.natlbcc.org

The coalition advocates increased funding for breast cancer research, improved access to high-quality breast cancer screening, diagnosis, and treatment, particularly for underserved and underinsured women.

- **National Comprehensive Cancer Network**
  50 Huntingdon Pike, Ste. 200
  Rockledge, PA 19046
  888-909.NCCN
  www.nccn.org

A nonprofit organization that provides reliable, specific, and easy-to-understand information for cancer patients, including Standards of Care and Treatment: Guidelines for Distress Management in Cancer Survivors.

- **National Health Information Center**
  P.O. Box 1133
  Washington, DC 20013-1133
  800-336-4797
  http://www.nhic-nt.health.org

This U.S. government agency aids consumers in locating health information.

- **National Lymphedema Network, Inc.**
  Latham Square
  1611 Telegraph Ave., Ste. 1111
  Oakland, CA 94612-2138

Provides referrals to lymphedema treatment centers, health care professionals, training programs, and support groups for lymphedema patients.

- **National Women's Health Network**
  514 10th Street NW, Ste. 400
  Washington, DC 20004
  202-347-1140
  www.womenshealthnetwork.org

This organization provides newsletters and position papers on women's health issues and concerns.

- **Native C.I.R.C.L.E.**
  The American Indian/Alaska Native Cancer
  Information Resource Center and Learning Exchange
  Charlton 6, Room 282
  200 First Street, S.W.
  Rochester, MN 55905
  877-372-1617
  www.mayo.edu/nativecircle

Resource center for providing American Indian and Alaskan Native cancer-related materials to health care professionals and the general public.

- **OMH: The Office of Minority Health**
  OMP P.O. Box 37337
  Washington, DC 20013-7337
  800-444-6472, 9 am to 5 pm EST
  www.omhrc.gov

The OMH maintains comprehensive databases on minority health issues and resources. Several OMH publications are available free.

- OncoLink—University of Pennsylvania Cancer Centre
  3451 Walnut
  Philadelphia, PA 19104
  www.oncolink.upenn.edu

A leading information Website developed and regularly updated by the University of Pennsylvania Medical Center Staff. The site has an extensive section on psychosocial support. Other sections include art, literature, video, poetry, performing arts, cancer and sexuality, coping, and spirituality.

- PISCES
  Partners In Self-Help Community Education and Support
  2021 Lakeshore Road, Suite 108
  Burlington, Ontario, Canada L7R 1A2
  905-637-2840
  www.pisces.on.ca

Leadership From The Heart is 2-day workshop providing skill development based upon the teachings in this manual. Programs can be delivered on site.

- SHARE, Self-Help for Women with Breast or Ovarian Cancer
  1501 Broadway, Ste. 1720
  New York, NY 10036
  212-382-2111
  212-719-4454 (Spanish)
  www.sharecancersupport.org

A self-help organization that serves individuals affected by breast or ovarian cancer. SHARE offers English and Spanish hotlines, peer-led support groups, public education, advocacy, and wellness programs.

- Sisters Network, Inc.
  8787 Woodway Drive, Ste. 4206
  Houston, TX 77063
  713-781-0255
  www.sistersnetworkinc.org

An African-American breast cancer survivor's organization involved in emotional support, research, cancer prevention programs, and advocacy efforts.

- **The Susan G. Komen Breast Cancer Foundation**
  5005 LBJ Freeway, Suite 250
  Dallas, TX 75244
  1-800-I'M-AWARE® (1-800-462-9273)
  9 am to 4:30 pm CST, Monday through Friday
  972-855-1600
  www.komen.org
  www.breastcancerinfo.com
  www.racenforthecure.com

The Komen Foundation is an international organization with a network of volunteers working through local Affiliates and Komen Race For the Cure® events to eradicate breast cancer as a life-threatening disease. The Foundation and its Affiliates fund research and non-duplicative, community-based breast health education and breast cancer screening and treatment projects for the medically underserved. The National Toll-Free Breast Care Helpline (1.800.I'M AWARE®), provides the latest breast health information. Se habla espanol. TDD is also available.

- **Y-ME National Breast Cancer Organization**
  212 West Van Buren St., 4th Flr.
  Chicago, IL 60607
  800-221-2141
  800-986-9505 (Spanish)
  www.y-me.org

Y-ME provides peer support and information to women and men who have or suspect they have breast cancer.

- **YWCA Encore Plus program**
  1025 Connecticut Ave., Ste. 1012
  Washington, DC 20036
  800-953-7587
  www.ywca.org

Encore Plus is a breast and cervical cancer outreach and screening program for women over 50.

Index

A

B

C

D

E

F

Living with Breast Cancer

G

H

I

J

L

S

T